The SECRET *to* LONG LIFE *in Your* DNA

The Beljanski Approach to Cellular Health

HERVÉ JANECEK, Ph.D.,
with MONIQUE BELJANSKI

Translated by Cheryl A. Metzger

Healing Arts Pres
Rochester, Vermont

Healing Arts Press
One Park Street
Rochester, Vermont 05767
www.HealingArtsPress.com

Healing Arts Press is a division of Inner Traditions International

Originally published in French under the title *Santé et Longévité par les plus récentes avancées médico-scientifiques issues des recherches de Mirko Beljanski* by Guy Trédaniel Éditeur, Paris
First U.S. edition published in 2009 by Healing Arts Press

Note to the reader: This book is intended as an informational guide. The remedies, approaches, and techniques described herein are meant to supplement, and not to be a substitute for, professional medical care or treatment. They should not be used to treat a serious ailment without prior consultation with a qualified health care professional.

Library of Congress Cataloging-in-Publication Data

Janecek, Hervé.

[Santé et longévité par les plus récentes avancées médico-scientifiques issues des recherches de Mirko Beljanski. English]

The secret to long life in your DNA : the Beljanski approach to cellular health / Hervé Janecek ; with Monique Beljanski ; translated by Cheryl A. Metzger. — 1st U.S. ed.

p. cm.

Includes bibliographical references and index.

Summary: "The first English presentation of the Beljanski method of fighting cancer from within the DNA"—Provided by publisher.

ISBN 978-1-59477-259-7

1. Cancer—Nutritional aspects. 2. Cancer—Diet therapy. 3. DNA. 4. Health.
5. Longevity. I. Beljanski, Monique. II. Title.

RC268.45.J36 2009

616.99'40654—dc22

2008044983

Printed and bound in the United States by Lake Book Manufacturing

10 9 8 7 6 5 4 3 2 1

Text design and layout by Priscilla Baker
This book was typeset in Garamond Premier Pro

The SECRET to LONG LIFE in Your DNA

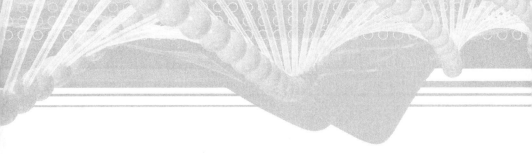

CONTENTS

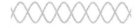

ACKNOWLEDGMENTS

I would like to dedicate this book to the memory of Mirko Beljanski (1923–1998), an exceptional researcher and pioneer in biology—one of the most prolific of the second half of the twentieth century.

My thanks go to Monique Beljanski, his wife, first of all for her presence, but also for her unwavering support and aid in the writing of this book.

I would also like to thank Sylvie Beljanski-MacCarthy, who has for many years tirelessly worked so that her father's legacy could be as useful and as accessible as possible to all those—and they are many—who might benefit from it.

Thanks also to those who have helped me by rereading, correcting, and enriching the manuscript of the book you now have before you. In particular I would like to thank Dr. Marie Haumont-Coolens, whose medical expertise and clinical experience inspired a good number of passages in this book. Her rigorous and precise approach to her patients has led her to use different medical techniques in combination with one another for several years now, which enabled her to discuss and correct this manuscript with authority.

Lastly, I wish to thank all of my close family members who have, with quite some patience, understood my absences and excused my distraction over the last year.

H. J.

USING THE ANTI-AGING STRATEGIES IN THIS BOOK

This revolutionary book introduces you to the groundbreaking work of the late Mirko Beljanski and his wife, Monique Beljanski. Their research and subsequent discoveries, undertaken in France in the second half of the twentieth century, led to the discovery of promising new treatments for cancer and other degenerative diseases.

Following Dr. Beljanski's death in 1998, the Beljanski Foundation was established in New York City by his wife and their daughter, Sylvie. A not-for-profit institution, the foundation was created in order to carry on Dr. Beljanski's work and to encourage and inform the world about his research.

This book, *The Secret to Long Life in Your DNA,* is intended to provide information to be used by the reader in conjunction with his or her doctor or other health care professional with the goal of attaining the best health possible. The material presented here—which makes it clear why an anti-aging strategy must be comprehensive—will support their effective collaboration. It is not intended to substitute for medical advice under any circumstances requiring consultation with a medical professional.

For anyone wishing to consult with a health care professional who is familiar with the Beljanski approach, please contact www.natural -source.com/engl/contact.php. To purchase the nutritional and supplemental products derived from natural compounds that Dr. Beljanski developed, please visit www.natural-source.com. However, with regard to the specific dosing for any and all supplements that are recommended in this book, please consult with a qualified health care professional. The author and his collaborators accept no responsibility for the use of the methods, products, or services proposed or mentioned in this book, nor for any damages, losses, or costs that the reader might directly or indirectly incur from their use.

To find further information about Dr. Beljanski and his discoveries and their seminal implications, please visit the foundation's website at www.beljanski.com.

FOREWORD

Michael B. Schachter, M.D., CNS

It is with great pleasure that I write the foreword to this unique book on anti-aging by Dr. Hervé Janecek. I have never met Dr. Janecek, so why am I writing the foreword to his book? I do so at the request of Sylvie Beljanski-MacCarthy, daughter of the biologist Mirko Beljanski, whose work is discussed in detail by Dr. Janecek.

Although I am a medical doctor and board certified in psychiatry, I have been involved with complementary and alternative (integrative) medicine for almost 35 years. Having used the Beljanski nutritional supplements with my patients since 1999, I am convinced that they are useful and helpful. As I have become more and more familiar with the life and work of the late Dr. Mirko Beljanski, I have also come to believe that he was the ultimate scientist and humanitarian, who I hope will some day receive the recognition and honors he deserves, albeit posthumously.

Thus, with great interest, I received Dr. Janecek's book. Modern medicine continues to struggle to help patients who develop cancer and chronic viral diseases, such as hepatitis C and AIDS. The most frequently used treatments for these conditions often have significant adverse effects and, in many cases, little potential benefit. As a result, complementary and alternative practitioners are constantly searching for innovative ideas and products that may help their patients, without causing undue side effects. With this in mind, I attended a conference in New York City in the summer of 1999 to learn about the work of the late Mirko Beljanski, Ph.D. I had never heard the name Mirko Beljanski before, but an old friend, the late Patrick McGrady Jr.—a well-known author and researcher who offered an information service called CANHELP for cancer patients—had urged me to attend. He assured me that I would learn some new things that could very well help my patients, so I decided to go.

There I learned that Professor Beljanski had been born in Yugoslavia in 1923 and at age 25 had emigrated to France, where he remained for the rest of his life. After completing his studies, he was accepted in 1951 as a biologist and researcher with the renowned Pasteur Institute. For almost 30 years he studied DNA and RNA and made numerous important discoveries. However, Dr. Beljanski was forced to leave the Pasteur Institute when his innovative ideas drastically conflicted with the institute's new director. Though underfunded, he continued his research and the publication of scientific papers, most of which were in French. He published 133 scientific papers during his lifetime. Tragically, he died in 1998 after several years of being persecuted in France for his groundbreaking work.

At the conference in New York I also met Dr. Beljanski's wife, Monique (who had worked with him in his laboratory for more than 40 years), his daughter Sylvie (who carries on her father's work by educating professionals and the public about his ideas, as well as running a nutritional supplement company that supplies products developed by Dr. Beljanski), and physicians, scientists, and patients familiar with Dr. Beljanski's work.

I was quite impressed with both the science presented in the lectures and the apparent benefits obtained by patients who were taking the products. Following the conference, I spent a great deal of time reviewing the material and began to use these nutritional supplements with some of my own cancer patients. Again, I was impressed with the results when incorporating the supplements into my work, which utilized a wide variety of complementary and alternative approaches, sometimes along with conventional treatment administered by surgeons, radiotherapists, and oncologists, and sometimes instead of these conventional approaches.

Reading this book gave me a deeper understanding and appreciation of the brilliance of Beljanski's original research and its practical applications. Though much of his research began decades ago, its importance is just beginning to be recognized in scientific circles. He developed concepts of cancer causation that allowed him to develop an important test, the Oncotest, for determining whether or not a substance is likely to cause cancer. This test is not being widely used yet, although it should be. Commercial interests help keep the technique suppressed, probably out of fear that many substances that are being used commercially would be shown to be carcinogenic and this would not be good for business. Of course, this is a shortsighted view; in the long run eliminating carcinogenic substances from our environment would be beneficial for the health of everyone and would also make wise economic sense.

Beljanski's theory about cancer causation also helped him to develop selective anti-cancer substances that suppress or control many types of cancer cells. This capacity was first demonstrated in test-tube situations and animal studies and then made available to cancer patients through Beljanski's work with doctors in France and Belgium. Many of these patients attest to their effectiveness. I myself believe that they have played a significant role in improving my results with alternative approaches to treating cancer.

Dr. Beljanski's contrarian notion that RNA could affect DNA, rather than just the other way around (the traditionally held view in biology), led to his conflicts with his bosses at the Pasteur Institute. But it is this discovery—which is now accepted in conventional circles—that allowed him to develop RNA "primers" capable of activating bone marrow stem cells. This important contribution has many practical applications, not the least of which is that cancer patients receiving radiation and chemotherapy can reduce their bone marrow suppression of white blood cells and platelets by taking these RNA primers. Recent preliminary results in research being conducted at the Cancer Treatment Centers of America have shown that these RNA primers can be extremely successful in preventing low platelet and low white blood cell counts, thus preventing the need for patients to prematurely stop their chemotherapy treatments.

Another practical application of Beljanski's work is that he found that a specific type of extract from the well-known *Ginkgo biloba* herb could reduce the activity of ribonucleases, enzymes that break down RNA and contribute to degenerative processes. This action of ribonucleases contributes to the formation of abnormal scar tissue (fibrosis), which is often seen when a person receives radiation for cancer. When patients take this special extract of *Ginkgo biloba* during or after radiation, fibrosis appears to be reduced, as evidenced by animal studies and the clinical reports of some patients.

Dr. Janecek discusses all of these concepts and phenomena in his book, explaining them in the context of biological theory. He also makes it clear that the observations of Beljanski may be beneficially applied not only for the management of cancer, but also in a wide variety of other clinical conditions, including viral diseases and autoimmune diseases like Hashimoto's thyroiditis and arthritis.

But Janecek's book goes beyond explaining Mirko Beljanski's work and its implications. He outlines a holistic and integrative approach to slowing down the aging process from many points of view. He is aware of the way in which the tissues evolve embryologically and how this must be considered in rebuilding and repairing the body. He brilliantly shows how the organism may be viewed as a hologram, with its component parts—the cells—containing the same essential elements as the organism itself. For example, he demonstrates that the nucleus of the cell is analogous to the brain and central nervous system of the organism.

In order to approach the problem of aging, he suggests that we must nourish and detoxify the cells, while also nourishing and detoxifying the organism as a whole. He offers some very specific suggestions for an optimal diet, emphasizing the role of high-quality proteins and fats and the optimal types and qualities of carbohydrates, vitamins, and minerals. High-quality food is the first order of business, but high-quality nutritional supplements should also be used. He discusses the role played by toxic substances, such as pesticides and toxic metals, in interfering with proper functioning of the organism at both the cellular and the organismic level. He suggests ways to reduce toxicity, including the use of chelation therapy to rid the body of toxic minerals such as lead, cadmium, and mercury. Exercise also plays a pivotal role in Janecek's approach to anti-aging, as this helps with oxygen utilization and detoxification.

Dr. Janecek believes that an anti-aging program should not deal with only one or two elements, but instead must deal with all elements simultaneously. Here he has brilliantly combined a general integrative anti-aging program from a holistic or holographic point of view with the ingenious work of Mirko Beljanski. The result is a stimulating and practical program that should benefit all readers who take it seriously.

MICHAEL B. SCHACHTER, M.D., CNS
MEDICAL DIRECTOR, THE SCHACHTER CENTER
FOR COMPLEMENTARY MEDICINE

Michael B. Schachter, M.D., CNS (Certified Nutritions Specialist), is the medical director of the Schachter Center for Complementary Medicine in Suffern, New York. The Schachter Center for Complementary Medicine was established in 1974 and is one of oldest centers in New York State to combine innovative ideas in nutrition and holistic health with the latest noninvasive developments in mainstream medicine. Treatment programs emphasize lifestyle changes and address diet, exercise, nutritional supplements, and stress management. For many patients, programs involving injectable vitamins, minerals, and chelating agents play a major role in treatment. Other modalities used include acupuncture and counseling or psychotherapy. Every effort is made to help patients embrace changes necessary to achieve optimal health. Several of the center's health care professionals have been on staff for more than 25 years. For further information about the center call (845) 368-4700 or visit the center's website: www.schachtercenter.com.

PREFACE

Monique Beljanski

I am grateful to Hervé Janecek for this remarkable book. In it I see the same rigorous reasoning and precise expression that have made him a very popular speaker in numerous European medical conferences in which I have taken part personally.

As the director of a biology laboratory, Dr. Janecek has for many years been familiar with the research that my husband and I have conducted. His familiarity with and intelligent grasp of our research places him in an excellent position to introduce his observations on the contribution of the "Beljanski strategy" to the optimization of body function when the aging process accelerates, and to do so in a form that a large public would understand.

The customary advice tendered in the "anti-aging" domain by those who have confiscated this extremely remunerative health niche is most often limited to methods for aesthetically masking the effects of aging. Meanwhile, access to publications concerning the degenerative ailments linked to aging remains too often the privilege of health professionals!

It is to the great merit of Hervé Janecek that he has highlighted in very accessible language the convergence of both the physiological and the environmental causes of deficiencies such as a lowered immune system, disturbed protein levels, chaotic cell growth, and so forth.

These deficiencies set the table for often terminal pathological conditions like cardiovascular diseases, diabetes, and cancer, but he demonstrates how they can be avoided, delayed, or arrested, thus beneficially paving the way for a dynamic and prolonged old age.

The strategy he advocates refers to the most recent advances in molecular biology and physiology and is supported by my husband's research performed at both the Pasteur Institute in Paris and our private CERBIOL laboratory. This strategy also is based on the use of the innovative molecules that we discovered, which are now the object of official clinical studies in the United States.

Monique Beljanski was born in Paris, where she studied biology and bacteriology before undertaking research in the field of molecular biology with her husband, the late Mirko Beljanski. This research continued for more than 20 years at the Pasteur Institute and yielded profound and significant contributions to the world of health and medicine. She worked for 10 years at the Faculty of Pharmacology in France and is retired from the National Center of Scientific Research in France. Monique Beljanski is the coauthor (along with her husband) of numerous peer-reviewed articles and the author and collaborator of three books that discuss the details and implications of their groundbreaking work. She is currently the president of the Beljanski Foundation (www.beljanski.com), which seeks to disseminate information about their findings and to encourage continuing research based upon their revolutionary discoveries.

FROM DNA TO OPTIMAL FUNCTIONING

Every living thing is born, grows up, reaches maturity, then declines, breaks down, falls ill, and dies.

We human beings are no exception to this rule. We often spend the first half of our lives preparing for and then earning a living in order to house, feed, and clothe ourselves, start a family, and live—or survive— only to face a mix of physical problems that handicap us during the second half of life, when we otherwise could have been enjoying a well-deserved retirement.

The passage of time and the wearing down of the tissues of the body that comes with it are unavoidable, but aren't there some ways to at least slow down this decline? With more people living longer than ever before in human history, this question is being intently asked by more and more individuals, and doctors and biologists, in ever increasing numbers, are attempting to answer it.[1] For many years now, the media has dedicated lengthy reports to various anti-aging strategies: products or methods having the specific goal of limiting the age-related damage or wear of cells, tissues, and organs. Most of the methods recommended are those considered to be truly natural, such as naturally sourced vitamin supplements or plant extracts. Natural anti-aging plans are favored because the public knows full well that prevention happens only over the long term, and only a nontoxic, natural plan to fight aging will be well tolerated over such a length of time.

However, it is not always easy to sift through the avalanche of recommended anti-aging solutions to determine which are of primary importance and efficacy. This book has been written to provide you with pragmatic, scientifically based guidance that treats the individual as a whole, integrating the microcosmic and macrocosmic perspectives, using the model of the hologram, in which each component reflects the whole.[2] It highlights nutritherapy, a short- and long-term therapeutic strategy that aims to progressively reestablish normal bodily functioning through food selection on the one hand and micronutrient supplements (such as vitamins, minerals, trace elements, and amino acids) on the other.

This book also highlights the pioneering work of biologist Mirko Beljanski, who, beginning in the 1960s, was one of the first to closely examine the ideal life of the normal cell, the multiplication of its DNA (the long molecules of deoxyribonucleic acid found in the cell nucleus, which is the seat of biological memory), and the various disorders that can occur.[3] This book presents—in simple, clear language—some of the essential findings of Beljanski's work, particularly those related to the negative impacts on human health and vitality that result from the destabilization of DNA and the amazing restorative capacity of RNA (ribonucleic acid).[4] His understanding of the specific mechanisms at work in the intimate biology of the cell enabled him to develop practical, simple, and ecological therapeutic methods for maintaining a healthy standard of living and preventing a number of degenerative illnesses—certainly the ultimate goals of every anti-aging method.

The anti-aging strategies presented here are based on the knowledge that certain principles of healthy functioning can be learned and beneficially applied. While the human body is complicated in appearance, it is simple in its organization, which can be viewed in terms of four principal, overall bodily functions:

- External protection (including assimilation and elimination)
- Internal structure and defense
- Energy production and distribution
- Memory and coordination

Clear understanding of these four functions offers important guidance for both preventing dysfunctions and reestablishing the innermost order of each cell and, more generally, of each individual. They can best be understood within a framework based upon a very simple description of the cell.

THE CELL: THE FUNCTIONAL UNIT

Cells are the functional units, the basic building blocks of all the tissues of the body.[5] Regardless of where they occur, cells share the same internal organization, which provides the basis for cellular functioning. Each cell is enclosed by an electrically charged membrane. This membrane is polarized, meaning that the external electrical charge is more positive than the internal charge (+/-); this causes the difference in electrical potential between the inside and the outside (see plate 1).

Within the cell membrane, the cell is divided into two areas: the nucleus and the cytoplasm. The nucleus, which is separated from the surrounding cytoplasm by another membrane, contains very long molecules of *nuclear* deoxyribonucleic acid or *n*DNA. DNA is the support structure for genetic information; particular segments of DNA molecules, known as genes, are responsible for specific functions in the cell (such as production of an enzyme, pigment, and so on).

DNA sends messages to the cytoplasm via RNA (ribonucleic acid). This *messenger* or *m*RNA is translated into proteins in the endoplasmic reticulum, the elaborate network of interconnected membranes that are continuous with the nuclear membrane. In addition to the endoplasmic reticulum, other small "organs" or structures, known as organelles, are present in the cytoplasm of every cell and are responsible for the day-to-day life of the cell. These structures, which handle digestion, cleansing, and defense, include the Golgi body (a group of flattened membrane disks found in the cytoplasm that digest and excrete numerous metabolites) and the lysosomes (vesicles present in the cytoplasm that are able to absorb foreign bodies and digest them using enzymes).

However, the most important role of the endoplasmic reticulum is the synthesis of proteins (such as various enzymes, support proteins, and hormones). In order to directly or indirectly ensure these different syntheses—which are needed for protection, digestion, and elimination—the endoplasmic reticulum is in a constant state of renewal. The reticulum remains in continual contact with the nuclear membrane, using ribosomes as intermediaries. The ribosomes, a type of organelle, occur on the surface of the reticulum and also move freely about the cytoplasm.

Nuclear DNA ensures the reproduction of the cell by dividing itself to create two identical nDNA. It can also break apart or become blocked, which leads to a disruption of its messages (degeneration) and ultimately to death of the cell (apoptosis).

Each cell owes its energy production to the mitochondria, little organelles present in large numbers in the cytoplasm that are capable of assimilating oxygen introduced by the blood. The mitochondria manufacture adenosine triphosphate (ATP) molecules, site of the biochemical energy of a cell. These ATP molecules also provide the electrical charges that polarize the cell membranes. In addition, they are the electromagnetic signals emitted and received by most of the molecules in the nucleus and the cytoplasm. Each mitochondrion also contains a molecule of DNA (*mitochondrial* or *mt*DNA) and is surrounded by a membrane, similar to the membranes that enclose the nucleus and the whole cell.

These central ideas about the life of the cell will make it easy for us to understand what is good for it or, conversely, to anticipate what will impede its healthy functioning.

DNA

DNA is a bit of a celebrity: it's talked about in the public as well as in the professional sectors; it is placed center stage in the cellular nucleus; and it contains the essential genes of the cell. Ever since the development of the assay to decode it, the notoriety of DNA has grown larger still. All the more reason, then, to know a little bit about how it works!

DNA is what we call a macromolecule, composed of two long chains of nucleotides. Each nucleotide consists of a sugar, one of four specific bases (abbreviated A, G, T, and C), and a phosphate group. The overall structure of the DNA molecule in space resembles a double helix. Although the two strands of the helix are continuously expanding and contracting, they are united by weak electrochemical forces called hydrogen bonds. Specific proteins, the histones, are in close contact with the DNA, serving as a matrix that provides support and protection for the double helix.

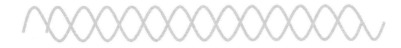

Fig. I.1. DNA is a chain of nucleotides presented in the form of a double helix.

At rest, the cell shows a three-dimensional DNA structure with a double helix and regular loops. When the DNA has to express itself—whether it be in order to synthesize proteins or for cellular division—particular enzymes (known as helicases) intervene, opening the double helix along its length. This makes all or several of the segments, the genes, available for transcription, in which an RNA copy of the genetic information in the DNA is generated.

First, the genetic information of the DNA is copied (transcribed) into messenger RNA. The mRNA then migrates into the cytoplasm, where it is translated into protein with the help of *transfer* or *t*RNA.

In DNA replication and cellular division, the DNA double helix is opened by enzymes in specific places to initiate the creation of its identical copy.[6]

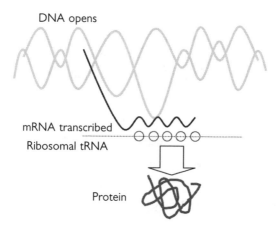

Fig. I.2. DNA opens, and messenger RNA is made and then translated into a protein.

Thus, whether for partial expression or full duplication, DNA opens its double helix, allows the necessary information to be expressed or duplicated, and then closes itself.

DNA is also subject to the phenomenon known as destabilization, caused by an attack of free radicals, carcinogens, or toxic substances. Such attacks can result in the partial opening of the double chain of nucleotides in several places, which can lead to problems in the life of the cell and ultimately to cell death. However, the long DNA molecule is continuously repaired by enzymes, themselves activated by trace elements. Our genes are thus well protected, but at the same time, they

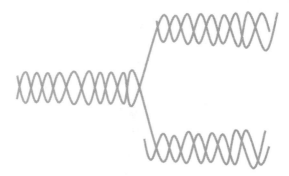

Fig. I.3. Production of two identical DNA from the initial DNA strand.

remain fragile, in constant evolution, and very sensitive to influence by elements in the cell's surrounding environment.

Behind the unique face of each individual lies his or her genetic makeup. While it is said that the expression of 30 percent of our genes cannot be altered, we estimate that we can influence the other 70 percent! This is evidenced by the extraordinary polymorphism observed among human beings (who share 99.9 percent identical DNA).[7] We thus have the potential to change a large part of our genes' expression through our nutrition, environment, and lifestyle. By using the information on the following pages, we can benefit from this plasticity, and actually influence the course of our lives . . .

FROM THE SINGLE CELL TO THE LIVING, WORKING BODY

Every human being is, at the beginning, a zygote—that is to say, a single cell, born of the fusion of a person's parents' germinal cells, or gametes, the ovum and sperm. The DNA of this egg continually divides over the next nine months in order to form the tissues and organs of the body.

This initial DNA from the egg is described as "totipotent," capable of synthesizing all the proteins for all of the cell types that make up the body's tissues. But as cell divisions take place and cells become specialized (differentiated) to form ever more specialized tissues (connective, osseous, musculatory, and so on), an ever-increasing portion of the genes that are able to be expressed in the egg are no longer able to be transcribed or expressed by the specialized cells.

DNA could be compared to a gene "library," in which all of the books are initially available to be read. Over time, however, as the differentiation of tissues progresses, first entire shelves are incrementally closed off, and then, within each book, entire chapters are sealed off one after the other.

The whole organism is composed of three principal layers of tissue: the endoderm, the ectoderm, and the mesoderm. The egg division first forms the ectoderm, which then forms the other two layers, all the while respecting an anatomical gradient between internal and external.[8] It also maintains an electric gradient: just as there is a polarization (+/-) between the inside of a cell membrane and its outer surface, there is a polarization between the layers of tissue.

The original three layers—the ectoderm, mesoderm, and endoderm—generate a total of six layers of distinct tissues (see plate 2). The ectoderm first differentiates the brain and nervous system tissue, then forms the endoderm, which produces the internal mucous membranes and a number of endocrine glands (such as the thyroid and thymus) and exocrine glands (such as the pancreas).

The third layer, the mesoderm, appears between these two layers. The mesoderm forms four layers. One layer, the bones and muscles, ensures the movement of the body; two layers, one composed of the arteries and the other of the veins and lymphatic vessels, ensure the transport of blood and bodily fluids; the final layer, the connective tissue and blood cells, constitutes the internal framework of the body.

The resulting structure of the body is a precisely assembled grouping in which all the tissues are arranged between the interior and exterior (see plate 3).[9]

These six layers of tissue are found throughout the body, where they form organs that are adapted to specific functions (such as the heart, lungs, liver, kidneys, stomach, and intestines). However, for the purposes of the discussion that follows, it is helpful to observe the concentration of the tissues of the three source types—ectoderm (1), mesoderm (2), and endoderm (3)—in the three main levels of the body: the head, the thorax, and the abdomen.

- At the *cerebral* level, the tissue is mainly of the nervous system—derived from the ectoderm (1)—including the brain, which imprints its rhythms (α, β, δ) on the rest of the body.
- At the *thoracic* level, the tissue is mainly circulatory—derived from the mesoderm (2a)—including the heart and lungs, which ideally synchronize in rhythmic, cardiorespiratory harmony.

- At the *abdominal* level, there are two main types of tissue: the mass of connective, sanguine, and lymphoid tissue (present everywhere, of course, but with a preponderance in the abdomen)—derived from the mesoderm (2b)—and the essential assimilation structures (stomach, intestines) and elimination structures (liver, kidneys)—derived from the endoderm (3).

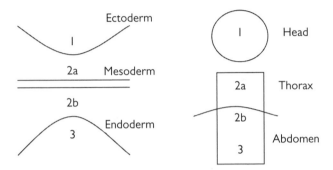

Fig. I.4. The concentration of tissue types in relation to three levels of the body.

Though it has since been substantiated by modern embryology, this three-part description of the body is not new, as doctors from ancient China—those who invented traditional Chinese medicine—described the person as composed of three stages: one stage facing the sky or Heaven and the exterior (which compares to the ectoderm and the nervous tissue); a second, intermediate level (which can be compared to the mesoderm and the connective, osseous, musculatory, and vascular tissues); and the third turned toward the earth and the interior (analogous to the endoderm and the mucous membrane tissue).

The body is not only a mass of molecules; it is information. Overall, the entire body remains polarized between the internal structures (the organs, blood, and connective tissues) and the external ones (such as the nervous system tissue, which includes the brain). The nervous system tissue retains the geography of all the parts of the body in its memory and supports the most intensive electric activity. Electrical exchanges between the brain and the rest of the body via the intermediary of the nerves, pervasive throughout, create a current flux in both directions. In the same way, the different flows of blood, both arterial and from the lymph, also create a strong longitudinal current of electrical charges.[10]

The ensemble of these fluctuations of particles, electrons, ions, and charged molecules makes up the amplitude of each individual's personal magnetic field.

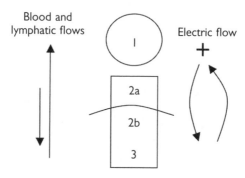

Fig. I.5. The constitution of the body's magnetic field: from the dynamic fluctuation of charges and electrolytes (charged molecules or ions) between the vascular centers (heart), nervous centers (brain), and their peripheries.

THE "HOLOGRAPHIC" MODEL OF BODY AND CELL

The three main tissue types have a direct correspondence to the four principal bodily functions (see also plate 4):

TABLE I.I

Source Tissue Layer	Tissue Type	Principal Function
I. Ectoderm	Nervous system	Coordination and memory
2a. Mesoderm	Circulatory (including heart and lungs)	Energy production and distribution
2b. Mesoderm	Connective, blood, and lymphoid	Internal structure and defense
3. Endoderm	Mucous membranes and derivative glands	External protection (including assimilation and elimination)

These four functions can be seen operating at the cellular as well as the whole body level.[11] Although the organs and tissues have different forms related to their respective functions, they are composed of the same basic units, cells, which recreate their functions on the microscopic scale (see plate 5).

1. Ectoderm

The DNA in the cell nucleus is analogous to the brain in the cranial cavity: like the brain, it is the seat of individual memory and the general coordinator, in this case of cellular activities.

2a. Mesoderm

The mitochondria in the cytoplasm find their match in the heart, continued by the arterial network: their activity is rhythmic like the organ itself. What's more, the mitochondria bring glucose and oxygen together in the cell to produce energy, which mobilizes all the cytoplasmic molecules. In the same way, the heart takes oxygen from the lungs and extracts sugar from the intestines in order to transport them together to the body's cells.

2b. Mesoderm

The multishaped network of the endoplasmic reticulum in the cytoplasm ensures the structure of the cell, giving shape and function (digestion, synthesis, nutrition, defense) to the majority of its organelles. Similarly, the connective tissue, of varying density, pervades the bodily tissue and organs, which the blood and the lymphatic tissues nourish and defend.

3. Endoderm

The external membranes and the endoplasmic reticulum correspond to the skin and the mucous membranes; mechanical and biological barriers, they make the decision as to what enters and leaves the cell. They are at once protectors, nurturers, and points of elimination.

TABLE I.2. FOUR FUNCTIONS AND CORRESPONDING STRUCTURES OF CELL AND ORGANISM

Functions	Cell Structure	Bodily Structure
Coordination and memory	DNA	Brain
Energy production and distribution	Mitochondria	Heart, lungs, arteries, veins
Internal support and defense	Cytoplasm and structural proteins	Bone marrow, connective tissue, lymphatic tissues
External protective barrier	Membranes	Skin and mucous membranes

The correspondence between the organization and function of the invisible and the infinitely small and that of the body as a whole can be helpfully understood in terms of a hologram: a three-dimensional image of an object or subject in which each part of the image is a reflection of the overall object. In other words, a hologram could be compared to a mosaic made up of pieces, each of which reproduces the entire mosaic in miniature; each piece examined under a magnifying glass would give a view that, although distorted, was faithful to the whole. (Please see the appendix, "Holography and Holograms," for a comprehensive explanation.) Although the 10^{13} cells of the body are not identical, they are like facets of a hologram, all sharing the same basic structural components and the same four principal functions seen in the body as a whole.

A COMPREHENSIVE ANTI-AGING PROGRAM

The anti-aging or preventive medicine model recommended in this book is new because it deals with both levels in the body, the macroscopic and the microscopic: the whole mosaic and each of its pieces (see plate 6). The strategies presented here treat the body as a whole—a hologram—an approach that yields much more rapid and consistent results and certainly more lasting ones.

This book calls for the synergistic use of strategies beneficial to cell and individual alike in order to restore normal vitality. It is clear that an anti-aging program—one that effectively compensates for the wearing down of tissues—must be comprehensive, taking into consideration both the three fundamental tissue types and the four main functions of the body. It would be useless to have mucous membranes in perfect shape to protect the body's borders but a brain that is compromised, or to have a nervous system in working order but limited core energy or nonexistent immunity. The functions and tissues are totally interdependent (see plate 7) and they must together be maintained in the best condition!

This program thus includes actions focused on the organs and their functions on a macroscopic level (such as the intestines and digestion, the heart and physical activity, the brain and memory), while at the same time including actions focused on improving functioning at the microscopic cellular level through molecular supplements.

It is the comprehensive nature of this anti-aging program that makes our approach truly scientific. What is of prime importance is the overall strategy, rather than a commercial product or two, even if those cited in this book are the results of extremely successful research and studies. The basic notions presented here will provide the basis for discussion and further exploration with a health professional. (There is a glossary at the end of the book to facilitate an understanding of the terms contained herein.) The reader, aware that implementing different complementary measures is not only possible but also advisable for maintaining health over the long term, can trust an experienced therapist for advice rather than looking to a laboratory—a person rather than a product. Presenting this new way of thinking and related information is the primary objective of the discussion in the pages that follow.

I

EXTERNAL PROTECTION, ASSIMILATION, AND ELIMINATION

As we have seen, the endodermic tissue that forms the lining between the exterior of the body and all the organs can be compared with all the cellular membranes that fulfill the same function on a microscopic scale. The mucous membranes—also called the border, assimilation,

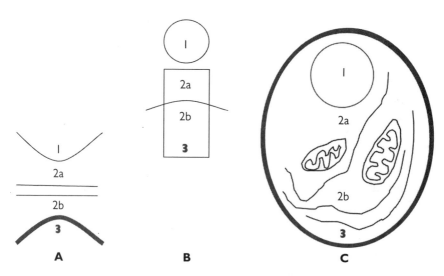

Fig. 1.1. The skin and the mucous membranes are analogous to the cell membranes.

and secretion epitheliums—form the essence of the body's internal lining: they constitute a mechanical barrier, and most importantly an extraordinarily fine biological filter.

Of the approximately 450 m² of these internal linings, more than 75 percent are the mucous membranes of the intestines and the organs connected with them (liver and pancreas).

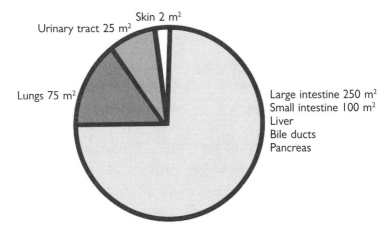

*Fig. 1.2. The mucous membranes of the intestines represent
75 percent of the body's internal lining.*

All of the mucous membranes fulfill two roles: assimilation (food in the intestines, air in the lungs, the re-assimilation of minerals in the kidneys) and elimination (intestinal or pulmonary secretion/excretion and renal filtration). In addition, the intestinal mucous membranes have an altogether unique status. At 1/40 mm in thickness, they are like a delicate parchment separating two worlds: the blood and the tissues on one side, and very active and numerous bacterial populations on the other (see plate 8). In fact, there are ten times more bacteria in the intestines than there are tissue cells in the whole body.

In order to age in good health, that is to say, in order to safeguard optimal tissue vitality despite the time that passes, it is important to:

- Facilitate consumption of quality nutrients (the role of the intestine) capable of being assimilated and capable of continuously reconstructing the elements being used by the body
- Facilitate the removal of toxic molecules, or those incompatible with the individual (the role of the liver and kidneys especially, but of the intestines as well)

This dual strategy implies ideal functioning of the mucous membrane lining in both directions, whatever the particular bodily region.

MALFUNCTIONING OF THE MUCOUS MEMBRANES

A healthy diet is essential for proper assimilation. On the molecular scale, the food we consume should contain proteins, nucleic acids, lipids, carbohydrates, vitamins, minerals, and trace elements. However, meals prepared these days are rife with numerous flaws; essentially, they contain too many "fast sugars," too many "slow sugars" (acid residue), too many saturated fats, and too much sodium (salt).

Importantly, today's meals also often contain too many indigestible, even toxic, molecules, which can include fat molecules turned into isomers (the *trans* or rigid form of heated oils caused by overcooking at excessively high temperatures), which cause chronic inflammation of the intestinal mucous membranes; amino acids altered by microwaving; and potentially carcinogenic compounds (such as Maillard proteins coming from glycation, frying oil teralenes, and the benzopyrenes of grilled meat).[1] Such altered molecules, absorbed daily for decades, constitute an important factor in aging.

Of course, this is without even mentioning pollutants, additives, and other industrial food preservatives. In addition, most often our meals do not have enough high-quality proteins, vitamins, trace elements, and phytonutrients from fresh fruits and vegetables (meaning they lack fibers and lipids) or enough unsaturated fats and potassium.

In the intestine, but especially in the liver and kidneys, the mucous membranes help with the reverse flow of undesirable molecules to the outside. If not for this, the body would create its own toxins, which would cause it to age much more quickly! The best way to prevent the onset of self-created toxins is, of course, through a healthy diet of well-prepared, fresh foods, whose different components are broken down by the digestive enzymes, aided by abundant intestinal flora rich in the bifidum bacteria particularly found in the colon. Following this ideal kind of digestion, nutrients are optimally assimilated and the body can easily handle any leftover elements.

Things do not always go so smoothly, however. What happens to food molecules can be divided into four possible scenarios:

TABLE 1.1

FOOD MOLECULE: ACCEPTED		FOOD MOLECULE: REFUSED	
1: Absorbed	2: Nonintegrated	3: Eliminated	4: Fixed
Growth	Clogging	Inflammation	Immune reaction
Maintenance	Cell asphyxiation	Skin and mucous membranes	Autoimmunity
Repairs	Intoxification		

If a food molecule has been accepted and the sugar or protein has entered the body and been absorbed (1), everything is going well; this is the fast track to differentiated growth and smooth physiological maintenance. This is also the path to healing and to general improvement.

But it is also possible for food components that are not likely to be beneficial to the body to pass the mucous membrane barrier (2). This is the case with overheated molecules (proteins, fatty acids), whose special configuration has been modified, making them unable to be absorbed. Instead, they wait to be burned up through oxidation before being broken into pieces and eliminated. This does not trigger an immune reaction, but the unabsorbed molecules are stored in the cells' cytoplasm, where they cause gradual clogging, which can, and often does, cause asphyxiation of the cell.

If the molecule is recognized as either foreign or harmful to the body, it can be eliminated through the skin or else through natural elimination organs, like the intestines, liver, or kidneys (3). This reaction is preferable and the mucous membranes, made more fluid through a natural wealth of unsaturated fatty acids, ensure proper elimination.

However, food-based and bacterial/viral protein molecules, which are external in origin, sometimes cross the permeable intestinal lining to join the intestinal flora before they are identified as foreign (4). Unfortunately, if such molecules are abundant and present in excess over time, they cannot be successfully eliminated. What's more, if they resemble the proteins found on the surface of our own cells, then our immune system, in attacking foreign proteins, will also attack our healthy tissues. This is what we call autoimmunity.

Clogging and autoimmunity both contribute significantly to aging. In both, undesirable foreign molecules result in the excessive stimulation of the organs assigned to their elimination; the kidneys are particularly vulnerable to deposits of undesirable complex molecules, which inhibit their elimination capabilities and facilitate premature aging.

The progressive deposit of undesirable molecules in the cells leads to cell asphyxiation and degeneration, as well as chronic intestinal infection, in which there is an imbalance of intestinal flora. With the abnormal development of putrefaction flora, high amounts of protein remnants called polyamines are released. While small amounts of polyamines are useful for stimulating the multiplication and maturation of normal tissues, they are harmful in large quantities. These extra polyamines paralyze nine-tenths of the immune system through cellular intervention.[2] Eighty percent of our stock of immune cells is found along the border of the intestinal mucous membranes (in the small intestine and colon); if there are too many polyamines from putrefaction related to bad bacteria in the intestine, then our largest source of immune potential, located behind the 1/40 mm thick intestinal mucous membrane, is not able to circulate.

THE NEGATIVE IMPACT OF FOOD INTOLERANCE

Our health is also negatively influenced by foods that are not well tolerated by our digestive systems. Intolerance to a particular food occurs when our digestive enzymes cannot break down the intruding molecule; if the structure of what remains after the enzymatic response is identified as foreign to the body, it first causes inflammation in the intestinal mucous membranes, and then, once the offending molecule has been absorbed and passed into general circulation, the inflammation may move into other tissues.

Tests largely developed in Europe (Great Britain, France, Belgium, and Germany) have made it possible to detect individual food intolerances through the addition of precise doses of immunoglobulin G to the blood. Immunoglobulin G (designated as IgG) is one of a class of proteins present in the blood and cells of the immune system that function as antibodies.

In the absence of such tests, it is difficult to precisely determine our food intolerances. However, Dr. Seignalet's research in France on wheat gliadins and milk proteins (lactoglobulins and casein) has shown that they may act as triggers for prolonging numerous autoimmune and clogging pathologies.[3] In addition, Dr. D'Adamo in the United States has shed light on the clear disparities in digestion potential as determined by an individual's blood group (A, B, O, or AB).[4] These differences concern:

- The overall volume of digestive secretions. The volume is higher for individuals in the O group, facilitating their digestion of animal proteins; it is relatively lower for those in the A group, who are more inclined toward vegetarianism.

- The compatibility of a given blood-type group with proteins (lectins) or surface sugars from food. This is seen most often through the salivary and digestive secretions.
- The composition of intestinal flora, whose different populations are inhibited or supported according to their proteins/surface sugars, which generally parallel those present in the different blood groups.
- The physiological variability of neurotransmitters (such as dopamine, serotonin, and nitrous oxide) in the different blood groups.

Even in the absence of individualized testing, the evidence for pathologies associated with modern wheat gluten and milk products, along with the indications provided by ABO dietetics, makes it possible for us to know which foods might be inflammatory. We can then review food ingredient labels to determine in advance whether or not a food poses the risk of causing a negative reaction or, to put it simply, whether it will be difficult to digest.

ANTI-AGING STRATEGIES TO AID PROTECTION, ASSIMILATION, AND ELIMINATION

Healthy aging starts first, year after year, with good nutrition, which can best be understood in light of the fact that proteins and essential unsaturated fatty acids construct and nourish our mucous membranes, ensuring their fluidity.[5]

Secondly, it consists of care for our digestive tract in order to avoid chronic inflammation, "leaky gut," and the imbalance of flora. Relieving the intestinal mucous membranes of persistent, chronic inflammation guarantees their relative impermeability to a good number of toxins and antigens (specific marker proteins), whether of food, bacterial, or viral origin.

Finally, it is important to spare our liver and kidneys, organs that specialize in drainage for the body. When the biliary tree and the renal collectors are encumbered with molecules that can be eliminated only after they are broken down by a complex and costly catabolic process, the remnants of that process once again generate inflammation and, therefore, general wear and destruction.

Five Questions for Healthy Nutrition

The most effective anti-aging strategy to aid the functioning of the mucous membranes to protect the body can take the form of five questions to ask yourself.[6]

- *Are there enough proteins on my plate?* An average adult should consume between 0.36 and 0.45 gram per pound of body weight, with special emphasis on high-protein foods (eggs, meat, fish, legumes, and complex cereals). For example, a person weighing 154 pounds should get between 55 and 70 grams of protein per day, primarily from fish, eggs, or meat, but also from legumes—over two meals—in order to continuously reconstruct the body's tissues, the base of which is actually the protein web.
- *Are the fats that I ingest each day of good quality?* The ideal is an equal proportion of unsaturated fats (fatty acid molecules that have a double or triple biochemical bond) to saturated fats (fatty acid molecules that do not have a double bond). Unsaturated fatty acids ensure an ideal fluidity in the membranes in all cells and their mitochondria, particularly in the brain, which has a vital need for long-chain fatty acids (like EPA, ecosapentanoic acid, and DHA, decosahexaenoic acid). Additionally, the unsaturated omega-6 and omega-3 essential fatty acids should be consumed in the ratio of 5 to 1.
- *Does my caloric intake match my physical activity?* Two thousand calories per day is considered the norm for an adult male, but each individual has his or her own optimal daily requirements, which vary according to the phase of life, amount of physical activity, season, and other factors such as pregnancy. Eating more calories leads to a faster metabolism (especially intestinal), more intense

agitation, and the at times dangerous interaction between sugars and proteins called "glycation," which results in AGE (advanced glycated end products), serious factors in the aging of all tissues. Also, if cellular respiratory capacity is exceeded, there will be more free radicals and lactic acid (see chapter 3, "Energy Production and Distribution").

- *Am I getting enough minerals, trace elements, and vitamins in the food I eat every day, not just for minimal functioning of my body but for optimal functioning?* Fruits and vegetables are rich in minerals, vitamins, trace elements, and the small metals that cause enzymes to work.

- *Finally, am I cooking, storing, and preparing food in such a way as to preserve its nutrients? Or am I leaching out nutrients, despite initially making healthy meal choices?* It is crucial to ensure what we call a "living" diet—rich in unprocessed foods that are eaten raw, steamed, or even lightly baked, one in which the foods are able to deliver nutrients.[7]

The practical answers to these five questions can be found in a diversified and balanced diet that one can calculate as to quantity and quality based on the pyramid on page 23; this diagram shows the types of unprocessed foods and their quantities to be absorbed each day.

Line **1** shows **one** serving of springwater per day, of 1 to 2 liters (about 1 to 2 quarts) or even more depending on the season, climate, and physical activity. The water should be purified, slightly acidic (with a pH between 6 and 7), and with an especially light mineral content.[8] It should preferably be nonoxidized, with an average oxido-reduction potential between 23 and 25. Water is important not for what it brings but for what it takes away: the inorganic mineral salts that are only very weakly digested in the intestines.

Line **2** shows **two** servings of proteins (of animal or vegetable origin, with a preference for fish and poultry over red meat), in sufficient quantity (about 0.4 gram per pound per day), especially for growing

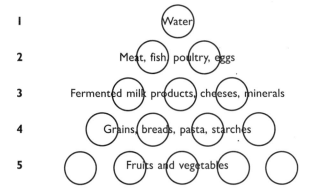

1   Water

2   Meat, fish, poultry, eggs

3   Fermented milk products, cheeses, minerals

4   Grains, breads, pasta, starches

5   Fruits and vegetables

Fig. 1.3. A diversified diet whose ingredients are distributed in the form of a pyramid diagram (adapted from Doctors Garnier and Waysfield).

children, pregnant women, menopausal women, and elderly people who tend to have more trouble with assimilation. Insufficient protein leads to fragile bones, a compromised immune system, and a lowered level of neurotransmitters and hormones, all of which cause premature aging.

Line 3 shows the need for **three** daily servings of foods rich in calcium, magnesium, and other minerals (iron, zinc, potassium). Insufficient amounts of these minerals result in fragile bones, lack of muscular force, permanent fatigue, diminished fertility and immunity, and limited cellular respiration. Three of these minerals deserve special mention:

Magnesium, the key element in immune and muscular contraction responses, is also indispensable in the respiratory cycle in mitochondria and in receiving cerebral signals produced by the synapses, the junctions between the neurons or nerve cells. Magnesium is found in abundance in green vegetables and dried fruits.

Zinc acts as a catalyst for more than a hundred different biochemical reactions. Major sources of zinc include seafood and dried fruits.

Potassium balances sodium (salt), which is often found in cooked meals and is frequently responsible for high blood pressure.

Eating organic potassium will not only lower blood pressure but also fight osteoporosis, because when the body works to expel excess salt there is a subsequent, lasting loss of calcium. Potassium is found in fruits and vegetables.

Those who are lactose intolerant or who have trouble with milk proteins should avoid nonfermented dairy products (cheese, cream, and ice cream). The 80 percent of the population that falls into this category, that is, the majority of people, can supplement minerals by eating lightly cooked fruits and vegetables.

Line 4 indicates that we should select **four** servings of foods rich in "slow" sugars, such as cereals, potatoes, bread, and so on. Slow sugars, sources of energy that are indispensable to the release of insulin—and thus to the healthy integration of proteins and fats—should be consumed at each meal. Even though we all need slow sugars, we must take care to eat only the amount of sugar that can be burned by the oxygen we inhale, and no more. In the long term, regular, quantitative caloric excess leads to obesity, resistance to insulin, and diabetes.

Line 5 refers to the **five** portions of fruits and vegetables that ideally should be eaten each day. Rich in phytonutrients, vitamins, minerals, and trace elements, these foods contain our natural antioxidants. However, fruits should be eaten outside of set meal times, and in relation to season: plenty during the summer, but very moderate amounts in winter (except for dried fruits). Body weight should also be taken into account (thinner people have more trouble than heavier people transforming fruit acids).[9]

Supplementing this "living" diet with cold-pressed virgin olive oils, nut oils, canola oil, or cameline (a plant of the cruciferous family cultivated in Europe) oil allows for the indispensable addition of unsaturated fatty acids to our cellular and mitochondrial membranes. Cold-pressed extracts contain fatty acids in the *cis* form, which makes them active, fluid, biologically available, and easy to assimilate.

Nutritherapy Recommendations

The following two nutritherapy strategies are also recommended to facilitate new construction and continuous repair of the mucous membranes:

- Nourish the intestinal flora by taking probiotics, an important source of several billion lactic bacteria, along with prebiotics, soluble fibers that accelerate their growth. They should be taken two or three times a week for several months at a time.[10] Regular supplementation helps to permanently sustain the bifidum flora responsible for maintaining the integrity of our intestinal mucous membranes and for the synthesis of vitamins, in particular group B, which supports healthy brain function.
- Provide border cells with the necessary fuel, including vitamin A and zinc, and particularly the amino acid L-glutamine.

Apply the 80/20 Rule

It is not necessary to make these suggestions into some new religion, but many years of experience in Europe show that this preventive diet leads to good health and can even be a weapon against a number of chronic diseases.

If we follow this advice for at least 80 percent of our lifetime or every day for at least 80 percent of the food that we consume, we will have a good chance of enjoying good health and vitality, and of enhancing the body's ability to repair itself.

If the proportion is reversed, however, health problems will emerge.

2

INTERNAL STRUCTURE
AND DEFENSE

The connective tissue formed by the embryonic tissue pervades the organs and reinforces the weblike structures supporting them. This diffuse mesoderm, present in all the tissues and organs, is analogous to the network pervading and differentiating the endoplasmic reticulum from the majority of organelles in the cytoplasm (such as the lysosomes and Golgi, as well as the peroxisomes, which enclose specific enzymes).

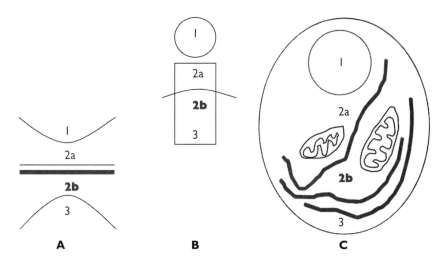

Fig. 2.1. The connective and lymphatic tissues are analogous to each cell's endoplasmic reticulum.

On the macroscopic scale, the skin and mucous membranes delineate the exterior shape of the body and constitute the borderline between internal and external, while the connective tissue gives form to all the organs by ensuring their framework and volume.

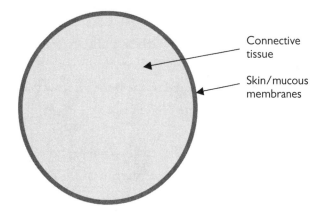

Connective tissue

Skin/mucous membranes

Fig. 2.2. The connective tissue supports the organs within the body.

THE IMMUNE SYSTEM

A particularly important derivative of the connective tissue is the lymphatic tissue, which monitors the body and its immunity in relation to fungi, bacteria, viruses, and foreign and degenerating proteins. This parallels the function at the cellular level of the endoplasmic reticulum, peroxisomes, and lysosomes, which are in charge of cleansing the cell and protecting it against intruders. Eventually, these organelles also digest and eliminate the internal structures that are no longer useful.

The majority of the lymphoid tissue (75 percent of its volume) is distributed just behind the intestinal mucous membrane lining, overseeing its 350 m^2 surface area. As a result of its proximity, the majority of the lymphatic tissue appears to be the reverse side of the whole mucous membrane surface. Like the mucous membranes, it is at once an entrance for nutrients, an exit for waste, and a tight and efficient barrier, as much as possible, against undesirable, external intruders.

But the cells of the lymphatic tissue are actually disseminated throughout the organs. These cells—which are mobile—come from stem cells, the cellular originators of tissue lines, located in the bone marrow. Bone marrow stem cells have a dual role: they form the basis of the blood cells and they can migrate anywhere and differentiate locally to match any cell type. They are described as being "totipotent" or "multipotent" because of their ability to transform into all cell types found in the body.

The stem cells located in the bone marrow generate five vital populations of red and white blood cells.

Red blood cells, called erythrocytes (1 in the diagram on page 29), ensure the transport of oxygen to the cells.

The four kinds of white blood cells are:

Leukocytes (2 in the diagram), the cleansing cells in localized action, are present in areas of inflammation (as polynuclear cells and macrophages).

Natural killer cells (3) are responsible, among other things, for eliminating cancerous cells.

B lymphocytes or plasma cells (4) produce large proteins (antibodies) in the blood called immunoglobulins, capable of fixing and neutralizing foreign proteins.

T lymphocytes (5), after maturation in the thymus and in collaboration with leukocytes, form the front line of protection against physical contact with aggressors (bacteria, viruses, cells with dangerous surface proteins, and so on).

Bone marrow stem cells, in addition to erythrocytes and leukocytes, are the basis for the body's defenses, whether the cells have a local action (T lymphocyte and cellular immune response) or whether they act at a distance (B lymphocyte and humoral immune response).

Recent studies have demonstrated that *stem cells have an extraordi-*

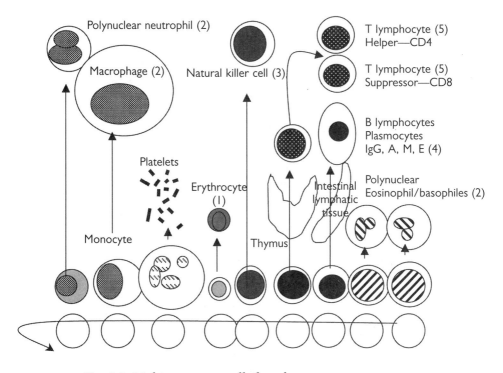

Fig. 2.3. Multipotent stem cells from bone marrow generate all blood cells and lymphatic tissue.

nary plasticity: they are in fact capable of settling, after migrating, into any tissue and playing a stem cell role in their new location, repairing local tissue, even in the case of cells that were considered to be unrenewable (such as nervous system and cardiac muscular tissue).[1]

Having a healthy immune system means that the body's capacity to classify and control external antigens and to determine whether the incoming antigens pose any danger is optimized.

An ideally functioning immune system responds to incoming food-based, bacterial, fungal, and viral proteins (with which we are always in direct contact) by accepting and tolerating those that are healthy and rejecting and neutralizing those that are not.

A person's immune system is rebuilt every day when he or she consumes an adequate amount of proteins (the immunoglobulins, spearheads of humoral immunity, are proteins), minerals and vital trace

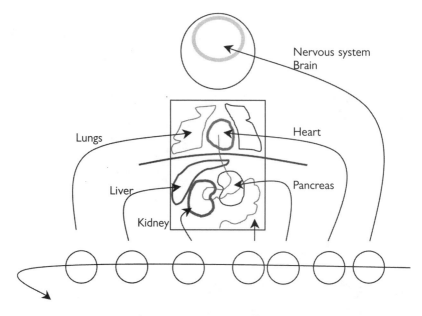

Fig. 2.4. Totipotent bone marrow stem cells are the localized repairers for all the tissues and organs.

elements like magnesium and zinc, vitamins like B and C, and, finally, polyunsaturated fatty acids, also called vitamin F. The latter ensure the fluidity of the cellular membranes and, therefore, allow for the mobility of the cells as well as their subsequent migration from one infection or inflammation to another.

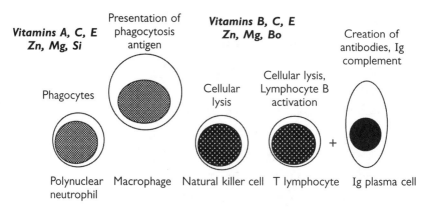

Fig. 2.5. The immune system is a bastion against potential internal and external aggressors.

MIRKO BELJANSKI AND RNA FRAGMENTS

We have seen that in the cell, DNA is like a library containing all genetic information. But what activates DNA, and what makes it enter into mitosis (the multiplication of the cell)? And, on the other hand, what are the factors that put DNA to rest or block it, thereby preventing it from working normally?

Biologist Mirko Beljanski (1923–1998) specifically studied DNA activity.[2] Many chemical factors, like hormones, can activate cell DNA through binding at specific sites. Conversely, poisons and heavy metals as well as gamma and X-rays are capable of damaging or even destroying DNA, either directly through a toxic action or through free radical intermediaries.

A little less than 40 years ago the experiments of Mirko Beljanski showed that DNA replication and hence cell proliferation could be both blocked and accelerated using tiny fragments of RNA.[3] Tiny segments of RNA (primer RNA) are capable of priming the division of normal cells,[4] while other RNA are capable of stimulating the division of cancerous cells at different sites. There are also certain types of RNA of specific lengths (antisense RNA) that are capable of hindering the division of cancerous cells or viral DNA.

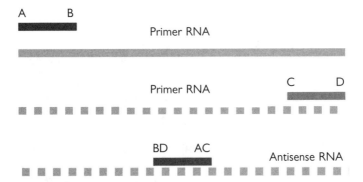

Fig. 2.6. Normal DNA stimulated by a primer (top). Cancerous DNA stimulated by another RNA primer of different length and sequence and at a different site (middle). Cancerous DNA or proviral DNA blocked by antisense RNA (bottom).

Mirko Beljanski was a pioneer in the therapeutic use of RNA. Beginning in 1975, in search of a means to reinforce the failing immune system of cancer patients undergoing chemotherapy or radiation therapy, he identified tiny RNA primers specific to bone marrow stem cells. He injected them into a severely immuno-deficient rabbit and found that these RNA were able, within 48 hours, to restore the rabbit's leukocyte population and platelet counts.

Likewise, for 25 years these tiny RNA primers have saved human lives by reestablishing the number of leukocytes, lymphocytes, and platelets in the blood, through the stimulation of the DNA of bone marrow stem cells. This has allowed thousands of patients to safely continue with their chemotherapy. These primers only weakly prime red blood cell precursors and so are not useful for treating anemia.

After the RNA fragments have served as primers, they are broken

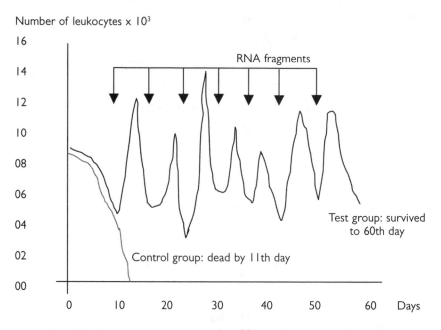

Fig. 2.7. Experiment in vivo with rabbits subjected to a lethal dose of cyclophosphamide (a chemotherapy molecule that directly acts upon DNA).

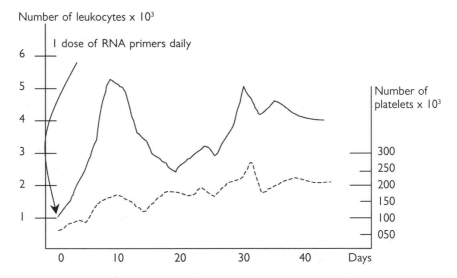

Fig. 2.8. Patient with lymphoblastic leukemia treated with classical chemotherapy and RNA fragments.

down into nucleic acid building blocks that can repair DNA damaged by radiation or chemotherapy products used in the treatment of cancer. Mirko Beljanski has also demonstrated this protective role for DNA structure.

Groups of mice that underwent radiation at 90 percent of the lethal dose for their species and size were also significantly protected by taking these RNA fragments. Moreover, in the five subsequent generations after this deadly radiation treatment, the young mice showed no phenotypical deficiencies visible on their bodies, reflecting the integrity of their parents' germinal cells and of the protection provided by the RNA fragments.

The results of Mirko Beljanski's experiments on antisense, antiviral, and anticancer RNA were reconfirmed in the 1980s by several American research teams.[5] The 2004 announcement in France by CNRS—Généthon d'Evry Laboratory—of a possible victory over the serious genetic disorder of myopathy through the use of RNA fragments was the logical follow-up to his pioneering work.[6]

In effect, biologists who practice gene therapy seek no longer to fully replace a defective gene, but rather to mask pathological DNA with antisense RNA fragments—without interfering with transcription of the remaining healthy genetic information. This little RNA is carried by a virus that enters the cell. The artificial infection it induces allows the antisense RNA encoded to the virus to be expressed.

The use of antisense RNA fragments to modulate—here, to mask—the activity of a defective, very precisely targeted DNA is once again generating interest in the study of the human genome for treatment of genetic disorders and perhaps also for the treatment of other types of degenerative diseases.

Even if today's researchers for the most part ignore the long and meticulous RNA research that Mirko Beljanski conducted more than 30 years ago, he can be considered to be the visionary forerunner of the most advanced biological technologies used today in genetic engineering.

STEM CELLS, THE NEW "EL DORADO" OF RESEARCH

Each tissue has differentiated cells within it that determine its function (such as muscle cells in muscles, pancreatic cells in the pancreas, and so on), along with stem cells, as yet nonspecialized, which are capable of replacing dead or injured cells. They are able to multiply and then adapt to fit the given need when the tissue or organ has been injured and needs replacement cells.

These stem cells exist everywhere, even in the nervous system. They resemble embryonic cells, still juvenile and without a real "job" until they are awakened. But bone marrow stem cells are special because they not only are capable of producing blood cells but also can migrate throughout the body, attach to a failing tissue or organ, and transform on-site into a healthy tissue or a specific cell.

Bone marrow stem cells are therefore able to do everything, or rather, to redo everything. This characteristic—useful even in nervous

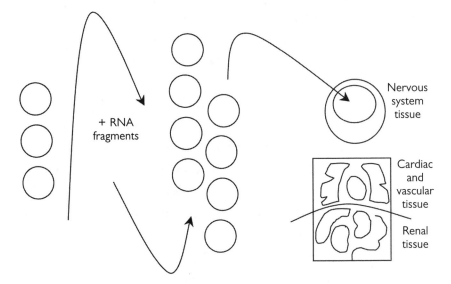

*Fig. 2.9. Multiplication of bone marrow stem cells by RNA fragments
for automatic cellular transfusion and repair of
various tissues and organs.*

system tissues or cardiac tissues that were long thought to be not at all
or only slightly renewable—is a recent and fundamental discovery.

A Canadian study at the University of Medicine in Ottawa has
shown that the administration of granulocyte colony-stimulating factor,
a growth factor in bone marrow stem cells, over 5 days to patients who
had undergone several myocardial thromboses allowed them to regain
a large section of their damaged hearts.[7] This experiment shows that by
stimulating bone marrow stem cell proliferation in vivo one can reconstruct a part of an organ, even one located far from the bone marrow
itself.

The demonstration of the ability of RNA primers to restore blood
cell supply to its optimal level supports the hypothesis that they can
at the same time facilitate the migration of a renewed supply of bone
marrow stem cells to an injured tissue or organ, allowing it to be
reconstructed on-site. Many clinical observations suggest that this is a
possibility; in fact, according to experiments conducted by numerous

doctors, these RNA fragments are able to reinforce the effectiveness of treatments for heart patients, those suffering from illnesses with functional impairment, and even those with degenerative nervous system diseases.

Unlike the growth factors used in the Canadian study, RNA fragments possess the invaluable capacity of self-regulation, which is imposed as soon as optimal physiological values have been achieved. They thus represent no concern regarding excessive stimulation of the bone marrow or overproduction of white blood cells or platelets. They cannot stimulate latent, possibly precancerous cells either, since the primer sites for multiplication of cancerous cells are different from the primer sites used in the reproduction of healthy cells.

Once introduced into circulation, these RNA fragments—which are of specific composition and length, and which are active on bone marrow stem cells—function like an army of micro-surgeons capable of recognizing signs of tissue wear and repairing the damage. They thus represent the perfect ecological means to fight aging by repairing and preventing organic dysfunction. This remarkable army of prevention is synergistic with the diet of micronutrients already cited, which supports the synthesis initialized by the RNA.

ANTI-AGING STRATEGIES FOR IMPROVING INTERNAL STRUCTURE AND DEFENSE

Protect Yourself with RNA Fragments

The immune stimulant and regulatory potential of RNA fragments is an invaluable advancement for anti-aging medicine. Their capacity to support optimization of the immune system and the body's subsequent production of stem cells can facilitate the regeneration of both organs and tissues. In order to realize this potential, I suggest that you take 1 dose of RNA fragments as prepared by Mirko Beljanski every week for 2 months, 3 times a year.[8]

The protective power of RNA fragments against radiation could be an added benefit to modern humans, who are now exposed to increasingly worrisome levels of electromagnetic pollution. In addition to the increased intensity of natural UVB rays due to the enlargement of the ozone holes at the earth's poles, we are exposed to medical X-rays, GSM cell phone emissions of electromagnetic energy, and Wi-Fi antennas. These antennas, located practically everywhere in our towns, are beginning to create a new danger, that of ELF (extremely low frequency) radiation, the long-term consequences of which (such as carcinogenic effects on living beings) no one can yet predict.

Therefore, taking these reparatory RNA fragments regularly is a good way to guard against new environmental aggressions. They should be taken in consistent treatments over the course of the year by all regular computer and cell phone users, as well as by all those who are passively subjected to relay antenna and wireless terminal radiations, which is to say practically everyone!

Remember Nutrition

Linking optimal nutrition with RNA fragments is a simple way to reinvigorate a weakened immunity. The nutritious diet recommended in chapter 1 to support healthy mucous membranes—one that is high in protein, polyunsaturated fatty acids, minerals, vitamins, and trace elements—is equally important for maintaining a good-quality immune system and the body's optimal capacity for self-repair.

So remember to consume sufficient protein (0.36 gram per pound per day); avoid foods that cause you to experience intestinal inflammation or trigger autoimmune responses, as they contribute to tissue wear; monitor your magnesium, selenium, zinc, and boron intake, as they are indispensable elements for the correct functioning of the immune response; and take supplements of essential fatty acids so as to maintain flexibility in the membranes of leukocytes and lymphocytes, cells that need to be mobile to be effective.

CASE STUDIES[9]

RNA Fragments and Immunity

Anne V.'s case is demonstrative of the potential for RNA fragments to stimulate immunity and regulation, even when the immune system is at its lowest. Her case demonstrates that priming healthy cell lines is possible even in the case of leukemia, because the location of stimulation sites in cancerous cell line DNA is different from the priming sites of healthy cell DNA.

Anne was born in 1964. In September 1981, at the age of 17, she began to suffer from chronic myeloid leukemia, which was treated with an antimitotic, Hydroxyurea. Two years later, in September 1983, her illness was uncontrollable and chemotherapy was no longer able to stabilize her white blood cells, whose numbers rose from 150,000 to 208,000.

At the same time, Hydroxyurea induced an extremely severe aplasia of red blood cells and platelets.

Both the clinic where she had been admitted and her father, who was a surgeon, agreed that she had only a couple of weeks to live and they decided to stop using Hydroxyurea.

However, at the end of September 1983, she began to receive 2 doses of RNA fragments per week; her platelet and red blood cell levels rose, which made it possible for her to start taking Hydroxyurea once again. This time it reinduced a decrease in white blood cells to 15,000 cells/mm^3 over three weeks.

The doses used were:

- 2 doses per week continuously at the onset
- 1 dose per month over the course of the remaining years

Anne lived quite comfortably for 10 more years while taking RNA fragments, demonstrating the protective potential of bone marrow RNA fragments when dealing with the sometimes useful, but often destructive, effects of chemotherapy.

RNA Fragments and Tissue Repair

The next case study demonstrates the potential of RNA fragments for inducing tissue repair within the central nervous system.

Nathalie L. was 44 years old in September 1983 and in the hospital when, after several debilitating bouts of an illness that were treated each time with high cortisone doses, she was diagnosed with multiple sclerosis.

The first time she went for a consultation was June 16, 1984; she had great difficulty with walking and supporting herself, coupled with leg weakness, pain, headaches, and a cold sensation in her foot.

Her treatment consisted of 4 acupuncture sessions and 3 doses of RNA fragments, taken successively at weekly intervals.

On July 23, 1984, she was able to walk 2 km and garden! She regained strength in her left hand and leg, the cold sensation disappeared, and she noticed a return to normal sensation. Her only remaining symptom was that her left thigh and leg were still painful to the touch. She took 2 more doses of RNA fragments in order to readjust to work.

By May 2004, 20 years later, she continued to do very well. There had been no worsening of her illness, and the gains she had made in 1984 remained. Over the 20 years, she took only about 20 preventive doses of RNA fragments, with no other treatment.

RNA Fragments and Immunity and Cerebral Development in Childhood

When the brain is still in the process of developing, it seems possible to rapidly enhance the connections being established between neurons (see chapter 4) via RNA fragment stimulation of stem cells, in such a way as to diminish disruptive childhood development problems.

Vincent V. was born in 1995 and lived with his parents in the countryside. In May 2001 his parents decided to consult a doctor after their child's behavior resulted in their being asked to withdraw him from traditional elementary school. It was recommended instead that they enroll him in a special school when classes began again in September. Essentially, Vincent demonstrated:

- Considerably slowed language acquisition: at 5½ he spoke like a child of 1½
- Hyperactive behavior
- Significant aggression
- Facial tics (1 or 2 times per minute)

He was treated with a single laser acupuncture session and his parents ordered RNA fragments; the protocol instituted was 1 dose every 2 days for 20 days, which began just 2 weeks after the May visit.

The child was next seen in October of the same year, at which point the parents explained that:

- The tics had disappeared after the acupuncture session.
- His slowed language acquisition, hyperactivity, and aggression progressively disappeared after 10 doses of RNA fragments.
- The child was able to return to normal schooling in September 2001. He did well academically in both semesters of his first year.

Jean S. was born in 1981. In December 1993, at the age of 12, it became clear that he was not adjusting well to regular schooling and he was at risk of flunking out.

His parents took him for a consultation. The child suffered from:

- Headaches
- Hyperactivity from anxiety and insomnia
- Tics of the head and hands, associated with cheek spasms
- Serious difficulties with concentration and memorization, which subsequently led to serious academic problems

During his childhood, Jean had been hospitalized 4 times for convulsions and he had had a bout of the shingles when he was 2 years old.

His first treatment, 2 sessions of acupuncture, yielded no results.

Beginning on January 18, 1994, he received 2 doses of RNA fragments per week.

- After 5 doses, he was already doing better.
- His tics, headaches, and hyperactivity progressively diminished.
- His academic problems significantly decreased and ultimately his academic status became normal.

3

ENERGY PRODUCTION AND DISTRIBUTION

In order to create an ample amount of energy, the body brings oxygen into the lungs from the air and transports it to the tissues via the erythrocytes in the blood, where it is enclosed by the vessels and propelled throughout by heart contractions. Finally it is absorbed into each cell, thanks to the mitochondria.

There are analogous structural, situational, and functional connections between the lungs and heart (and the major blood vessels situated

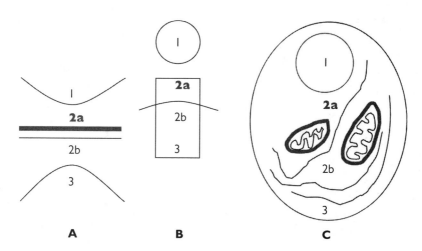

Fig. 3.1. The lungs, heart, and blood vessels are analogous to each cell's mitochondria.

at the center of the thorax) and the mitochondria located in the cellular cytoplasm: although at two different scales, both gather oxygen and nutrients, with the ultimate mutual goal being the synthesis of energy.

ATP AND THE KREBS CYCLE

The lungs, heart, and major vessels of the thorax (arteries, veins, and lymph vessels), built by the mesoderm, regularly contract in rhythm: 60 cardiac contractions and 12 full breaths (inhale/exhale) per minute on average. They are located in the center of the thorax, between the brain (the neurosensory center and general coordinator) and the abdomen (the metabolic center and the area where assimilation and elimination take place).

At the cellular level, the mitochondrion is the organelle in the cytoplasm that is itself the source of rhythmic contractions, the basis for ongoing changes in shape based on the need to create energy. Just as the heart is located in the center of the thorax, the mitochondria are located in the cytoplasm between the nucleus, the other organelles, and the exterior membranes. They retain a piece of DNA from their bacterial ancestor that allows for the local synthesis of enzymes and proteins that are essential to respiration.

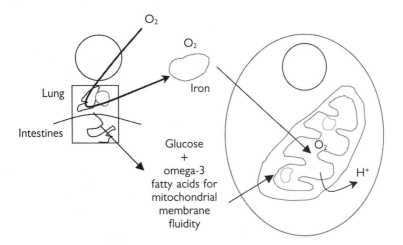

Fig. 3.2. From the lungs to the mitochondria, via the erythrocytes.

The function of mitochondria is to assimilate the oxygen brought to them via the lungs. Through the process known as *aerobic metabolism,* oxygen and glucose are transformed into carbon dioxide, water, and energy, called ATP or adenosine triphosphate.[1]

As ATP is the principal currency of biochemical energy in the cell, the processes responsible for creating it are essential. In addition to aerobic metabolism, there is also the process of *anaerobic metabolism,* which takes place in the absence of oxygen, in the cytoplasm outside of the mitochondria.

Although both processes share the same initial sequence of reactions, aerobic metabolism continues with the process known as the Krebs cycle to produce far more energy: 36 ATP molecules compared with only 2 from anaerobic metabolism.

All tissues and organs benefit from this source of energy, the liver and brain in particular. The latter consumes 20 percent of the body's glucose and oxygen, while it weighs only 1/50 of the body's

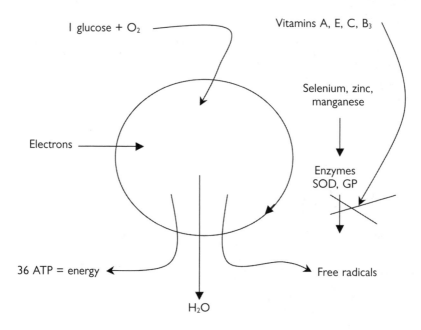

Fig. 3.3. The Krebs cycle in the mitochondria.

total weight: it is therefore 10 times more greedy for oxygen than the other tissues! This production cycle works only if the cell has certain nutrients at its disposal, like vitamins A, E, C, and B_3, minerals like iron and magnesium, and trace elements like zinc, manganese, and selenium.

THE THREAT OF FREE RADICALS

In addition to energy, water, and carbon dioxide, the Krebs cycle also generates oxygen radicals. While residual oxygen radicals are useful (they play an antiviral and antibacterial role within the lysosomes), they can also cause damage when they are produced in large numbers and not well neutralized by enzymes.

These free radicals attack the membranes and DNA (mitochondrial and nuclear) by oxidizing the fatty acids in membrane phospholipids and by breaking the weak bonds connecting the DNA bases in the double helix. This damage is responsible for notable aging of the cells. Indeed, it seems that the different signs of aging—premature or not—are caused by the accumulation of micro-lesions induced by free radicals, which occurs when the cells are unable to repair the lesions quickly enough.[2]

Mitochondrial membranes and DNA are directly exposed to free radicals, but some very simple substances are able to protect them by continually neutralizing free radicals in significant quantities and initiating repairs on exposed structures. Numerous studies have shown that the association of two micronutrients—acetyl L-carnitine and alpha-lipoic acid—can remarkably improve the physical and mental performance of elderly and lethargic rats.[3] The application of this work in human subjects, in particular for people suffering from degenerative neurological disorders, has been realized by a number of clinicians.

Acetyl L-carnitine facilitates the transport of fatty acids in the mitochondria, where they are converted into acetylcoenzyme A, which is directly used in energy production. Alpha-lipoic acid is an antioxidant, present in the mitochondria, that regenerates vitamins A, E, and C through biochemical reduction; neutralizes heavy metals like mercury; recycles coenzyme Q10, an essential product in the aerobic cycle; and normalizes the peroxidation of lipids.

The mass creation of ATP by the mitochondria (several kilos per day!) also allows for the production of S-adenosyl methionine (SAMe), a compound that is at the heart of fundamental biochemical processes. It is capable of methylating (that is to say, adding a unit of methyl to) biomolecules,[4] which is a means for the cell to neutralize the products that it is trying to discard while at the same time creating new essential fatty acids and peptides. This dual role of purification and synthesis is essential to the main cleansing organs like the liver, and also for the brain, an organ that lives only through the ongoing creation and neutralization of its neurotransmitters (SAMe is essential to melatonin synthesis starting with serotonin).

SAMe is also required for the synthesis of glutathione, a component of the key enzyme in the fight against free radicals, glutathione peroxidase. An abundance of SAMe makes it possible to effectively fight free radicals. On the other hand, a small amount of SAMe means there are fewer possible methylations, making it difficult to reconstruct the lipids and proteins necessary to bodily metabolism. This, therefore, means no healing and no repair, which leads, quite simply, to premature aging and death.

SAMe in turn requires the sulfur amino acid, L-methionine, and ATP, that is to say, more proteins and correctly assimilated oxygen. SAMe synthesis, particularly in the brain, is blocked by an elevated level of homocysteine (a peptide resembling two amino acids, cysteine and methionine) in the blood, a sign of premature vascular aging. However, folic acid, vitamins B_{12}, B_6, and B_9, and trimethyl glycine are able to correct an overabundance of homocysteine, recycling the methionine and making it possible for SAMe to be produced once again.

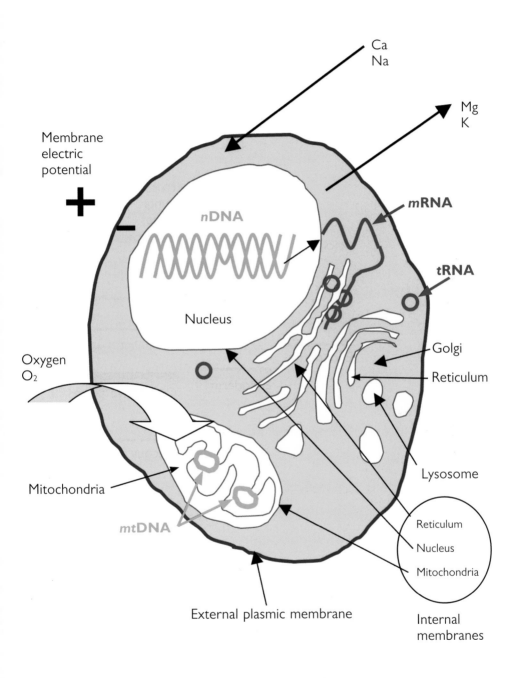

PLATE 1
Diagram of a basic cell.

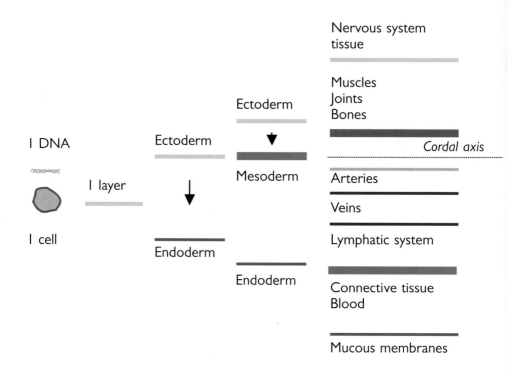

I DNA

I cell

I layer

Ectoderm

Endoderm

Ectoderm

Mesoderm

Endoderm

Nervous system tissue

Muscles
Joints
Bones

Cordal axis

Arteries

Veins

Lymphatic system

Connective tissue
Blood

Mucous membranes

PLATE 2
From the single cell to the multicellular being:
the formation of six layers of tissue.

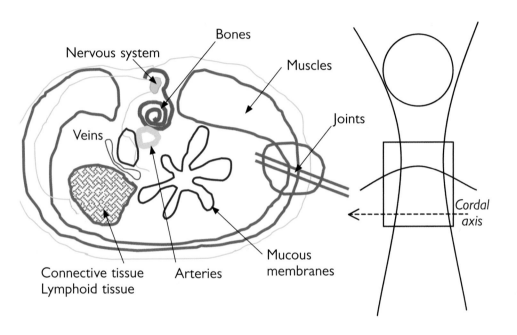

PLATE 3

Cross-section of torso: the six layers of tissues.

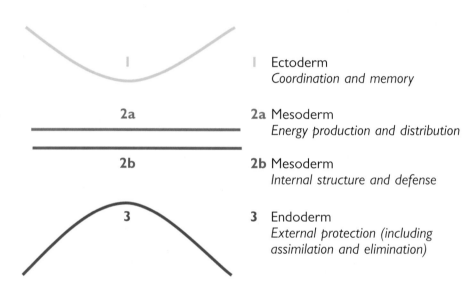

| Ectoderm
Coordination and memory

2a Mesoderm
Energy production and distribution

2b Mesoderm
Internal structure and defense

3 Endoderm
External protection (including assimilation and elimination)

PLATE 4
Three embryonic layers of tissue, four principal functions.

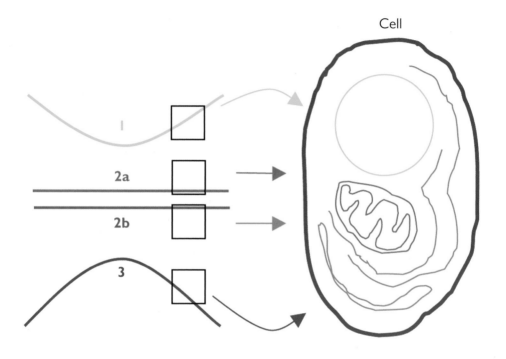

Cell

PLATE 5
*Three tissue layers and four functions of the
cell and organism.*

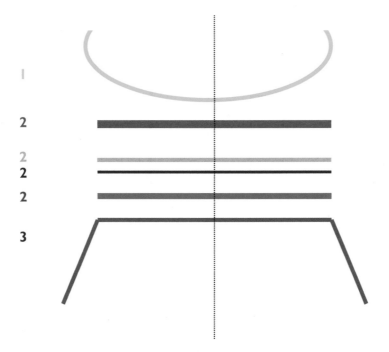

PLATE 6

Traditional Chinese medicine has already observed that
the body is built on a base of three different elements.

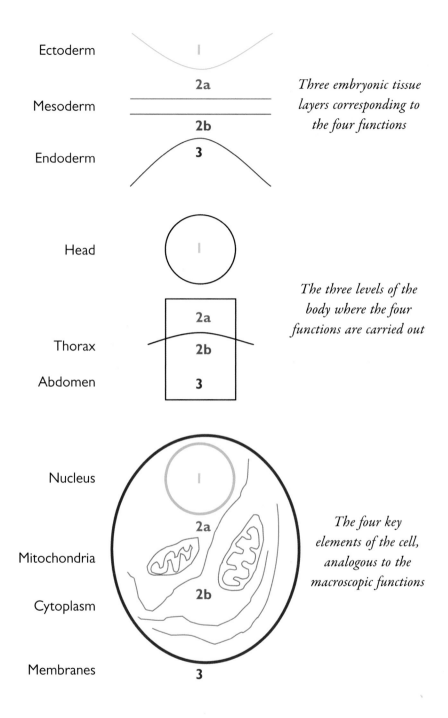

Ectoderm

Mesoderm

Endoderm

Three embryonic tissue layers corresponding to the four functions

Head

Thorax

Abdomen

The three levels of the body where the four functions are carried out

Nucleus

Mitochondria

Cytoplasm

Membranes

The four key elements of the cell, analogous to the macroscopic functions

PLATE 7

A holographic view of the body, wherein the cell represents the facets of a hologram and share the three-level structure of the body and its four functions.

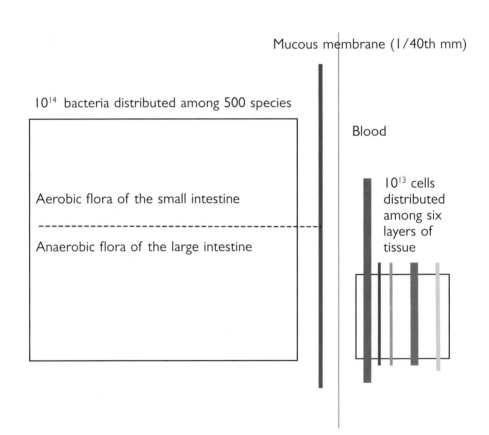

Mucous membrane (1/40th mm)

10^{14} bacteria distributed among 500 species

Aerobic flora of the small intestine

Anaerobic flora of the large intestine

Blood

10^{13} cells distributed among six layers of tissue

PLATE 8

The intestinal mucous membranes—1/40 mm in thickness—separate a gigantic bacterial universe from the blood that bathes our tissues.

Clearly, free radicals and the accumulation of noncatabolized molecules within the two fundamental structures of the cell—the membranes and DNA (particularly in the mitochondria)—are significant risk factors in physical decline. These factors worsen with age and are exacerbated by a diet deficient in protein, vitamins, and trace elements.

SUGAR AND AGING

If the amount of calories (sugars, fats) consumed exceeds the amount of physical exercise, then not enough oxygen is available to burn them up. They are then processed by the anaerobic pathway outside of the mitochondria, producing only 2 ATP per molecule of glucose, instead of the normal 36, along with a robust production of lactic acid.

An overall excess of fast and slow sugars in the blood gradually leads to a biochemical process called glycation, a damaging reaction of sugar, protein, and oxygen, particularly in the proteins associated with DNA and the membranes. Accumulation of glycation molecules in the cell is associated with several age-related diseases, including diabetes, Alzheimer's, cardiovascular disease, and cancer.

Glycosylation, the enzymatic addition of a sugar to another molecule, is a major source of aging in proteins. It can be prevented with a low-calorie diet and by taking carnosine (or beta-alanyl-L-histidine), a dipeptide capable of preventing both glycation and free-radical-induced oxidation.

With age and decreased energy, the natural and essential breakdown of oxidized proteins by proteasomes (protein complexes) begins to falter, as it is based on a reaction requiring a lot of energy (ATP).[5] Unfortunately in addition to being increasingly unreliable, this phenomenon also leads to the buildup of glycated proteins in the system. In light of this, prevention yet again proves to be vital.

HEAVY METALS VERSUS
GOOD ENZYMES

Another danger to the Krebs cycle, the major producer of our cellular energy, are the heavy metals, such as lead, cadmium, aluminum, and mercury. These metals are found in city air—because of cars and factory discharges into the atmosphere (lead)—in cigarette smoke (cadmium), and in vaccines and dental amalgams (aluminum, mercury).

These heavy metals have the ability to block the enzymes that function in the respiratory cycle by substituting for necessary trace elements like selenium or zinc. In place of the trace elements, they attach themselves to the center of enzymatic molecules, including those that are essential to the neutralization of free radicals or to repairing DNA.

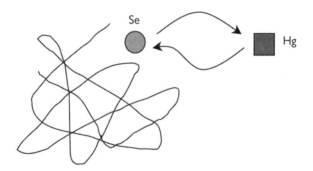

Fig. 3.4. Mercury replaces selenium within an enzymatic molecule, rendering the molecule unable to function.

For example, in the presence of mercury, glutathione peroxidase (GPX) is deprived of the selenium that it needs in order to function. Without glutathione peroxidase, there can no longer be an effective anti-radical defense. Numerous free radicals will no longer be neutralized, leaving them free to attack membranes and the cellular DNA.

Avoid exposure to heavy metals whenever possible, as aging of the tissues goes hand in hand with an accumulation of heavy metals and free radicals and a reduction of trace elements in the cells. However, if inhaling or ingesting these heavy metals cannot be avoided, there are ways to encourage their removal. Heavy metals can be chelated, that is to say, isolated, in the tissues where they are found (brain, liver, skin, mucous membranes, and so on) and purged through salts or urine.

Certain natural products—including fatty acids, amino acids (taurine), certain essential oils, and aromatic plants like garlic and coriander—facilitate the removal of heavy metals, even from the nervous system. Vitamin C is also able to facilitate the removal of heavy metals like lead and mercury. Injectable and oral EDTA (ethylene diamine tetracetate), a synthetic amino acid, is also a chelating agent useful for removing lead and cadmium.

ENZYMES OUT OF CONTROL

As the body ages, the connective tissue becomes increasingly damaged due to the buildup of free radicals and changes in the operation of enzymes, particularly collagenase and elastase. Collagenases break the chemical bonds between the molecules of collagen, the main protein of connective tissue and the most abundant protein in the body. They play a protective role by destroying extracellular structures such as bacteria that target the connective tissue in muscle cells and other body organs. However, when collagenase is overproduced, it can cause fibrosis, the formation of excess fibrous connective tissue.

The enzyme elastase plays a similar role: it breaks down elastin, an elastic fiber that, together with collagen, determines the mechanical properties of connective tissue. Like collagenase, it has positive functions and, when overproduced, can lead to dysfunction.

The overproduction of these enzymes leads to degeneration: healthy, functioning cells are gradually replaced by fibroblasts while sclerosis of the tissues sets in. Fibrosis gradually takes over the endocrine glands, bone marrow, muscles, small vessels, articulations, and, more generally, connective tissue. Pervasive fibrosis becomes a major obstacle to the delivery of nutrients to the tissues.

In chronic inflammatory illnesses such as hepatitis, arthritis, and thyroid and pancreatic autoimmune diseases, this process is accelerated and parenchymas (the functional parts of the organs) age all the more in the process of ossifying. Severe fibrosis is also caused by therapeutic radiation; it is linked to the activity of free radicals that are mass produced when radiation waves hit the cell.

Yet another enzyme that can "run amuck" is ribonuclease, which catalyzes the breakdown of RNA. It is capable of selecting RNA at specific sites, enabling the cell to use RNA primers for new multiplications, but in the case of cancer, this process must immediately be halted.

A Special Ginkgo Extract

While conducting research into molecules able to combat the overproduction of these enzymes, biologist Mirko Beljanski became interested in *Ginkgo biloba*, a major antioxidant in the world's pharmacopoeia.[6] Rich in terpenes and flavonoids, ginkgo has been used for centuries for its anti-radical properties and ability to facilitate cerebral oxygenation. But Beljanski discovered that it offered other wonderful benefits.

From the golden yellow leaves of the ginkgo tree, he selected a complex of acids with mildly anti-radical properties. Produced by a unique extraction/purification method from only the golden leaves of the ginkgo tree, the Beljanski Ginkgo V extract shares just 3 percent of its molecules with the popular green leaf extract. Beljanski found that this particular golden-leaf ginkgo extract is a powerful enzyme regulator. When ribonuclease is produced in excess, for example, the extract has the ability to slow down the continuous priming of mitosis in a cancerous or proviral cell.

Moreover, the ginkgo extract also proved to be a collagenase inhibitor. This has been demonstrated by its strong antifibrosis capacity, in most tissues and organs, though it appears to work especially well with

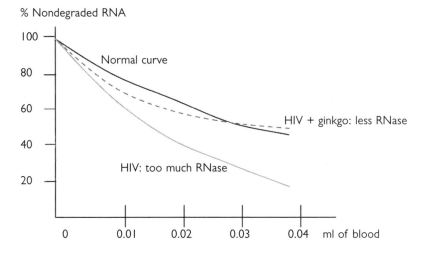

Fig. 3.5. Chart of ribonuclease (RNase) inhibition over four years in an HIV patient taking the Beljanski ginkgo extract in order to fight enzymes like ribonuclease. The top line demonstrates a normal curve, the middle line demonstrates the effect of ginkgo, and the bottom line demonstrates an abundance of ribonuclease in an HIV patient not taking the extract.

the liver, the brain, and the endocrine glands. Cancer patients undergoing radiation therapy have been able to avoid (or minimize) burns and the severe fibrosis usually caused by the radiation by taking the Beljanski ginkgo extract during treatment.[7] The proven ability of this ginkgo extract to reduce or stop fibrosis of all types illustrates its value as a major anti-aging product.

Furthermore, it has been shown that this golden-leaf extract diminishes the rate of hepatic transaminase (another enzyme) in the case of chronic viral infection and degeneration, which leads to cirrhosis of the liver.[8] The Beljanski Ginkgo V extract, in conjunction with other antioxidants like vitamins A, E, C, and B_3 and zinc, selenium, magnesium, and manganese, helps restore optimal local oxygenation, without oxidation.

Finally, this extract effectively treats heavy metals, which activate uncontrolled DNA multiplication.

ANTI-AGING STRATEGIES FOR OPTIMUM ENERGY PRODUCTION AND DISTRIBUTION

In order to optimize cellular energy production, combine several of the following effective strategies:

- Create your own energy through daily moderate exercise (such as walking, biking, gymnastics, and so on) that works every part of your body. If possible, include exercise in your workday in order to economize time and make it unavoidable.

- In addition to choosing a living diet, rich in fruits and vegetables with a sufficient intake of vitamins, minerals, and trace elements, adapt your caloric intake to your daily physical expenditure in order to avoid any exaggerated instances of glycation.

- To specifically fight against free radicals, take vitamins A, E, C, and B_3 and zinc, selenium, magnesium, and manganese, which could be considered "first degree" antioxidants. Vitamin C also protects connective tissue by inhibiting enzymes like collagenase.

- Take L-carnosine, a dipeptide that is particularly able to prevent the glycation of histone molecules in DNA.

- Protect mitochondria and DNA with acetyl L-carnitine, which facilitates the transport of fatty acids burned as energy in the mitochondria, and with alpha-lipoic acid, whose role is to regenerate glutathione, itself the originator of glutathione peroxidase, the key enzyme in the respiratory chain. Acetyl L-carnitine and alpha-lipoic acid are antioxidants that qualify as mitochondrial protectors.

- Facilitate the detoxification of dangerous and encumbering molecules and promote cellular anabolism by having an abundance of SAMe, an essential methylation product. Direct supplementation is essential if the body is sick and if a tissue or organ is degenerating.

- As needed, chelate heavy metals with specific natural techniques, including intake of selenium, sulfur, and aromatics. Some aromatic plants with these benefits are actually quite common, like garlic, which is rich with sulfur and selenium, and coriander. A detoxification strategy is usually carried out for several months, and sometimes even several years.
- Use the Beljanski Ginkgo V extract to help regulate enzymatic activity. It will aid the catabolism of senescent cells, thereby eliminating excessive metals, and reduce fibrosis associated with age, thus freeing up cells to function optimally.

With regard to the specific dosing for any and all supplements recommended in the list above, and any and all supplements suggested elsewhere in this book, please consult with a qualified health care professional.

CASE STUDIES

Anti-Fibrosis Ginkgo

Nicole B., born in 1928, was suffering from infectious hepatitis that had developed into cirrhosis. On July 14, 2003, an ultrasound of her abdomen revealed splenomegaly and hepatomegaly (increased size of the spleen and liver) and irregularities in the left lobe of the liver. There were signs of hypertrophy of the portal vein and fibrosis. A daily regimen of 5 Beljanski ginkgo gel caps over a 6-month period was undertaken, resulting in steady improvement in liver enzymes and platelets over time, as shown in table 3.1.

In addition, an ultrasound of the liver in March 2004 showed that the patient's cirrhosis had stopped progressing. From the beginning of treatment, the patient felt "more alive" and said she was "happy to be living."

TABLE 3.1. NICOLE B. CASE STUDY

	Norms	July 2003	March 2004	June 2004	Nov. 2004
Platelets x 10^x	150–450	97	118	129	151
SGOT (aspartate)	<34	87	83	55	30
SGPT (alanine)	<44	92		57	45
γGT (gamma glutamyl transpeptidase)	<36	297		208	42

Patrick E. was born in 1942. He was operated on for hemorrhoids in October 1996, at the age of 54. Unfortunately, the first surgery was complicated by severe narrowing of the rectum and anus, which required that the surgeon perform several intestinal colostomies and plasties between December 1996 and March 1997: the anal opening was so constricted that the surgeon was able to examine only 2 mm in depth, while the narrowing extended for 10 cm.

The patient's first consultation was in July 1997 for depression, due to two failed attempts to fit him with an artificial anus to reestablish a normal passageway. The surgeons no longer dared to operate.

A protocol of 5 ginkgo gel caps per day was begun. Two months later the stenosis had become much more flexible and a dose of RNA fragments was added, to be taken every 5 days on an empty stomach.

In March 1998 the surgeon, seeing the obvious improvement in the basin sclerosis, agreed to operate again. He was able to reestablish a normal anal passage. Since that day, no complications have arisen and no narrowing has been found.

Ginkgo and Arterial Hypertension

Born in 1934, Jean H. developed high blood pressure in 1970. In 1985, he suffered an acute episode of pulmonary edema (fluid collected in his lungs) and his blood pressure dropped.

In 1999, he once again suffered an acute edema of the lung following a coronary thrombosis. Upon examination of the cardiogram, a serious, almost total narrowing of the coronary arterial network was visible, with the impossibility of angioplasty by dilation and the impossibility of a coronary bridge. His surgeons proposed a coronary bypass surgery, which the patient refused. Doctors predicted that without bypass surgery, he wouldn't live more than 6 months.

He began taking 5 ginkgo gel caps per day and 2 doses of RNA fragments per week. In 4 months, his overall condition was transformed. He recovered from his severe shortness of breath and was able to once again go out, work on various projects, and even buy a house. An echocardiogram revealed that the left ventricular hypertrophy had disappeared!

4

COORDINATION
AND MEMORY

The brain is the vital center of the body, the seat of individual memory, the place where all the activities that occur in the body are recorded and regulated on several levels. It should, therefore, come as no surprise that its nutritional and energy demands are much higher than those of any other tissue.

Because cellular memory is stored in the cell's nuclear DNA, it makes sense to compare memory of this kind, encrypted in a succession

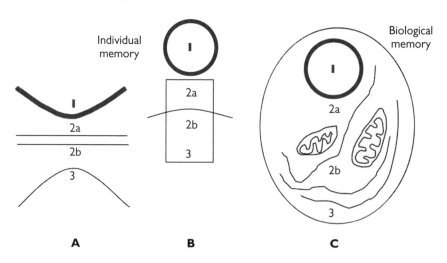

Fig. 4.1. The brain is analogous to nuclear DNA.

of DNA bases, with that of the brain, which houses individual memory and records it into the neuronal synapses.

At a macroscopic level and at a cellular level, the brain and DNA together constitute the fourth—and highest—level of functioning in the body: the one responsible for coordination and memory.

Like every other tissue, the nervous system as a whole is composed of cells. There are three types: gray-matter neurons, white-matter oligodendrocytes, and astrocytes present in supporting tissue. These three types of cells originate from the neuronal stem cells, which independently reproduce near the cerebral ventricles.[1] They reproduce in the hippocampus, the area of the brain essential to memory, and then migrate to the areas where they may be of use.

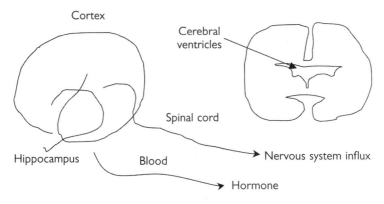

Fig. 4.2. The brain and the cerebral ventricles.

The nervous system sends and receives messages. The neurons are famous for being the action cells of the nervous system; to transmit information they use both the electrical impulses along the length of their axons as well as chemical neurotransmitters and hormones, found locally or elsewhere in the body.

When a neuron's transmitted output reaches a target, the target responds in kind, stimulating the release of a responsive signal (such as a hormone or neurotransmitter; see left diagram on page 58) or an action (muscle contraction, eye movement, or thought process).

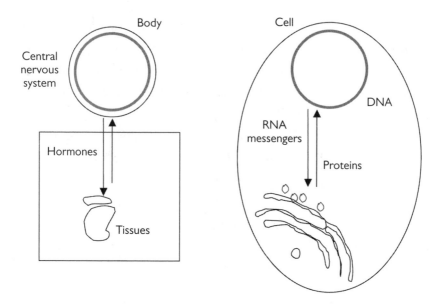

Fig. 4.3. Hormones and neurotransmitters are the messengers between the brain and the tissues (left) in the same way that, in a cell, RNA is the messenger between the nucleus and the cytoplasm (right).

On the cellular level (shown above at right), DNA acts in almost an identical way: it influences life in the cytoplasm via messengers, circulating and returning DNA or RNA.[2] In return, it is modified by other products whose creation it initiated (proteins).

RNAs are the messengers for DNA, just as the neurotransmitters and hormones are the messengers for neurons. Thus the techniques for protection on both levels are analogous.

A HEALTHY BRAIN FOR OPTIMUM MEMORY

As a whole, the neurohormonal axis—consisting of the brain, spinal cord, and hormones—constitutes the nucleus and the active elements of the "human" cell. When it comes to aging, physiologists and therapists rightly focus their attention on the brain's healthy functioning as indispensable.

But the brain is a fragile organ. It breathes 10 times more than other tissues and organs (except the liver); it is susceptible, like the other organs, to pollutants, catabolic waste, food-based proteins, viruses, and bacteria. Despite the relative protection of the meningeal barrier, it is also often afflicted with chronic inflammation, which results in the beginning of asphyxiation and degeneration of the tissue.

Problems with memory are often the first recognizable effects of neural degeneration that, in time, can compromise the health of the brain. A good memory presupposes above all that the cerebral structure remains healthy. Thus, in order to protect the neurons, it is not enough to "exercise" them by playing bridge, building models, going to conferences and concerts, playing an instrument, or even being active in a volunteer organization. Such basic cerebral activities do indicate that the neurons are interacting with each other. However, they do not indicate whether the structure that is storing all new information is in working order and remains coherent and healthy.

Our hypothesis, validated by research on memory, is that the structure where the brain stores information—in fact, the entire memory of the individual—is the thin film formed by neuronal synapses, the connections between neurons. Each neuronal cell contains a form of biological memory within its nucleus in the form of DNA. A membrane of connections is formed between these cells; in the crucial learning

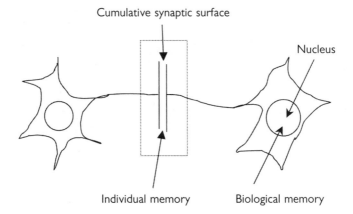

Fig. 4.4. The two types of memory: individual and biological.

zone of the hippocampus, where stem cells renew the supply of neu-rons, they continuously weave themselves a new cellular network. These new surfaces form an untouched lipido-protein synaptic film that can be compared to a constantly expanding holographic plate, a model that helps explain the brain's prodigious capacity for storing information on such a tiny physical surface.

Our hypothesis holds that in order to weave and renew this "holo-graphic plate"—the synaptic film structure supporting memory in the brain—our neurons have to function at optimal capacity. If the neurons degenerate or are renewed too slowly, the synaptic connections between them will degrade and the individual's memory will fade. Keeping our neurons healthy is thus vitally important.

One of the important ways to nourish our neurons is through the reg-ulated oxygen intake that takes place when we engage in moderate physi-cal activity. Deep breathing stimulates the rhinocephalus, one of three regions in the brain that produces new neuronal stem cells. Breathing more deeply thus has a direct effect on the ability to repair the brain!

Research on the optimal coordination of respiratory and cardiac rates (nicknamed "cardiac coherence")—brought about through men-tal relaxation—suggests that it is comparable to the electric influxes in the brain, otherwise known as the synaptic messages.[3] These boost the body's magnetic field, which coordinates the overall body's internal and external energy exchange.

Even more than other tissues, the nervous system needs high-quality proteins in order to construct itself. In addition to being used to build and rebuild connective tissue and to consolidate the membranes, proteins are required to produce cytokines (signaling proteins such as interferon and interleukins) and neurotransmitters (like dopamine, serotonin, acetyl-choline, adrenaline, and noradrenaline). Food-based proteins are also used to reconstruct new DNA (L-glutamine, an amino acid, is its essential precursor).

Though at first it may seem unnecessary to reiterate the importance of protein, a recent experiment illustrates that this message is still quite pertinent. We conducted a study with participants who were living in a supposedly wealthy country. In that study, we found that 80 to 90 percent of the participants, in all age groups, did not have enough protein—in terms of both quantity and quality—in their diets (0.36 gram/lb/day from eggs, fish, fowl, and meat).

As discussed in chapter 1, the quality of protein to be consumed is of vital importance: in order for a protein to be broken down into amino acids in the digestive tract, it must be recognized by our enzymes. The molecules of proteins that have been modified by overcooking become indigestible. In addition to the problems noted in chapter 1, these modified proteins can become models for pathological proteins, capable of externally generating abnormal proteins (like prions) or in any case altered peptides. The aging cell has increasing difficulty removing these altered molecules via the proteasome channel.[4]

The accumulation of beta-amyloid protein in the neurons, one of the signs of Alzheimer's, could be due in part to one or several of these irregular catabolic processes.

ANTI-AGING STRATEGIES FOR COORDINATION AND MEMORY

The way to protect the nucleus of any cell is through its DNA, the guardian of memory. This in turn is the way to protect the brain, the vital center of the body and basis of neurohormonal functions. Ideally, an anti-aging program targeting cerebral health should, at the very least, include a revolving combination of all the following basic nutrients and practices for optimal long-term vitality, in addition to moderate daily exercise.

- To protect the brain, as well as the kidneys, liver, and so on, against compounded pathologies, start by consuming functioning proteins that are raw or lightly cooked (cooked at a temperature not exceeding 230°F). The emphasis on including an adequate quantity of high-quality protein should start as early as possible and continue throughout life, since growing adolescents rely so heavily on protein and seniors have increasing difficulty absorbing and incorporating protein into their tissues.

- Polyunsaturated fats are also important to the brain, since 20 percent of its mass is composed of complex lipids like cervonic acid (produced starting with EPA). Both the flexibility and the vigor of the synaptic "holographic plate" are directly related to this portion of fatty acids. The sources of these fatty acids are vegetable oils (sunflower and flaxseed oils) and fish oils (EPA and DHA). These molecules are invaluable to the vitality of the neurons and their synapses.

- Figuring among the sources of lipids that are useful for memory are certain lecithin fractions, like phosphatidyl serine. Numerous studies have raised interest in the systematic intake of lecithin fractions for prevention of, and to supplement treatment for, memory problems.

- The brain is a major consumer of glucose and oxygen and, ideally, a major producer of energy in the form of adenosine triphosphate (ATP). At any given second, in order for its operations to be carried out, it requires the vitamins needed for aerobic life—vitamins A, E, C, and B_3—and associated trace elements—magnesium, zinc, manganese, and selenium. These nutrients prove all the more useful as the brain is increasingly saturated over a lifetime with toxic heavy metals, like gasoline lead and the mercury present in certain fish and especially in dental amalgams (see chapter 3).

- The protection and regeneration of these first-degree antioxidants with metabolites like acetyl-L-carnitine and alpha-lipoic acid is even more critical for the brain than for any other organ or tissue. S-adenosyl-methionine (SAMe), methylation agent and subsequent protein synthesizer, is also a powerful agent for regeneration in the aging brain.

- The practice called cardiac coherence, which connects breathing with visualization, helps control the energy flow that runs through the brain and heart. Mental and spiritual activities such as meditation can activate cardiac coherence.

HORMONES AND NEUROTRANSMITTERS
FOR HEALTHY AGING

It is now well known that micronutrients alone are not the only way of approaching the problems of aging. Hormones like steroids (DHEA, progesterone, and testosterone), growth hormones, melatonin, and thymic hormones, as well as neurotransmitters or their precursors, are employed to stimulate, repair, and regenerate tissues, especially those related to cerebral functions in the aging individual.

Several studies show that the quantity of neurotransmitters and hormones decreases with age, which has led biologists and doctors to use hormone supplements or their precursors with success in various ways.

Estrogens and Progesterone

The most widely distributed hormones taken today are without question synthetic estrogens and progesterone used in what is known as hormone replacement therapy. These hormones are prescribed to counteract the undesirable symptoms of menopause (hot flashes, vaginal dryness, loss of libido, and osteoporosis) and the signs of aging in women by

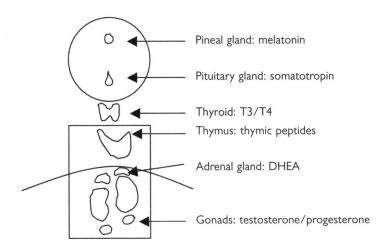

Fig. 4.5. Some examples of the main hormones produced by different glands.

attempting to compensate for the notorious drop in female hormones that begins between the ages of 45 and 50.

This cocktail of synthetic hormones has proven effective in the short term against clinical signs of menopause. However, over the long term it has been shown to be aggressive toward the very tissues that it is supposed to protect and revitalize. Recent studies conducted on more than 10,000 women undergoing hormone replacement therapy show a significant—almost 25 percent—increase in the risk of developing breast, uterine, or ovarian cancer compared with those not taking hormones.[5]

With age, the immune system is weaker and toxic environmental factors begin to accumulate, so the risk of site-specific cancer development due to a sometimes excessive hormonal intake is quite real.

This risk is significantly reduced if estrogens are avoided and natural progesterone (actually a semi-synthetic derived from yam) is used in their stead. Best administered on the skin in cream form, applied daily, it is recommended for avoiding the problems of osteoporosis, obesity, lowered libido, and so on faced by menopausal women. It appears to be a good solution to aging among women 45 and older, much more so than hormone replacement therapy with synthetic hormones.

Numerous plants (such as soy, chasteberry/monk pepper, sage, and alfalfa) can also be effective in treating postmenopausal symptoms by modulating estrogen and progesterone receptors.

Testosterone

Men also experience hormonal decline after age 50 to 55. This is known as andropause. Symptoms include fatigue, depression, gradual loss of muscle, a loss of libido, and erectile dysfunction. For this syndrome, testosterone, normally produced by the testicles as well as the adrenal glands, has been used with some success as a replacement therapy. The problem, however, is that imposing a fixed, daily dose of hormones on an aging body—in men as well as in women—poses an increased risk of cancer development. The natural tendency of prostate tissue to become cancerous, another age-related trait, can be exacerbated when testosterone is converted to estrogens.

In order to avoid the direct use of hormones, numerous phytotherapy solutions have been tested, among which the best known is the intake of extract of the root of *Tribulus terrestris,* known as caltrope or puncture vine, which is able to inhibit—by stimulating 5-α reductase—the aromatization of testosterone to estrogen.

DHEA

DHEA is one of the most abundant hormones in our bodies, produced by the adrenal gland and also by the nervous system cells in the brain. The amount of DHEA produced by an individual is a good marker of biological age. This is why replacement DHEA, made from soy or yam nuclei (which have a similar structure), has been recommended to reduce various signs of aging.

Moreover, since DHEA is an intermediate stage in the production of sexual steroid hormones, it increases the amount of estrogens, progesterone, and testosterone in the blood of those taking DHEA supplements. This hormonal increase is in physiologically normal doses, with the body producing only what it needs on its own and no more, a much more intriguing prospect than imposing doses by direct supplementation.

In animals as in humans, DHEA is capable of:

- Stimulating the enzyme that mobilizes L-carnitine in the liver (thus playing an anti-obesity role)
- Protecting the heart and the vessels by decreasing the accumulation of platelets and by reducing cholesterol
- Inhibiting a key enzyme in cancer progression, glucose-6-phosphate desaturase
- Directly inhibiting free radicals
- Restarting the cerebral physiology, which is a major anti-aging action

- Increasing bone density by stimulation of osteoblasts, which has major anti-osteoporosis effects
- Regulating immunity, particularly the autoimmune syndromes[6]

For people who have been diagnosed with low levels of DHEA in the blood, DHEA supplementation may be recommended, all the more so if the levels of progesterone and testosterone are also low.

Growth Hormone and IGF1

The youth hormone *is* the human growth hormone (HGH), but does that mean that it needs to be readministered to those who have low levels and want to be made young again? Signs of deficiency in HGH include pronounced biological aging, a loss of muscle mass, a weakening of the connective tissue, bone compression, and marked obesity. If all these signs are present, direct supplementation with HGH could be a way to treat this syndrome, but there is the danger of uncontrolled proliferation in stimulated tissues, which must be constantly monitored by medical professionals.

A promising alternative can be found in nutritional methods. One method in particular involves strong first- and second-degree antioxidants, a cocktail of precursor amino acids such as L-glutamine, glycine, and arginine, and a relatively low-calorie diet, which facilitates the adapted production of the growth hormone (GH) somatotropin and a revival of cerebral activity.[7] This regimen makes it possible to restore normal levels of IGF1—the growth factor produced by the liver, which is the principal marker for HGH activity—a direct consequence of the renewed growth hormone secretion the regimen initiates. Prescribing HGH no longer becomes necessary.

Thymic Hormones

The brain has many thymic hormone receptors, whose direct action is not yet understood. The thymus contains more than 20 different hormonal fractions (such as thymuline, alpha 1 thymosine, and thymopentine),[8] some with immuno-stimulant properties, and others with immuno-suppressive properties. Supplements containing these hormonal fractions have a recognized anti-aging effect; they have traditionally been used in northern and central Europe (Germany, Switzerland), but also in the United States and Canada. Like other hormones, they are as strong and effective as medications and must be prescribed in conjunction with other measures. It should be noted, however, that not all thymic hormone preparations are equal, as shown by research in Germany.

Melatonin

Melatonin is found in every animal species, and even in vegetables. It acts like an orchestra conductor arranging the other hormones. Dictating the sleep cycles of the brain with respect to external light, melatonin is perhaps the most important of all hormones. It is made by the pineal gland, a small gland located on top of the brain, which atrophies with age. Melatonin is derived from serotonin (whose precursor is the amino acid tryptophan).

The direct antioxidant action of melatonin explains why it is potent as an anti-aging supplement. Oral intake of melatonin has been tried as part of various strategies aimed at restoring cerebral function and different hormonal secretions. The problem is that the hormone is quickly destroyed in the blood; thus, the oft-recommended dose of 2 to 5 mg of melatonin to be taken in the evening 15 minutes before falling asleep is not necessarily good in the long term.

An alternative is taking an extract of bergamot, a plant that contains 5-methoxypsoralen (5-MOP), which stimulates the release of melatonin from the pineal gland. When taken in the early evening, this extract initiates the secretion of an effective, lasting dose of melatonin during the night. Regular intake of bergamot, along with the trace element zinc and S-adenosyl-methionin (SAM-e itself is absorbed in the morning), is a very powerful and perfectly biological anti-aging strategy.

Antioxidant Strategy for Hormone Production

Before quickly resorting to a regimen of high-dose hormone therapy, with the attendant risk of cancer, consider an antioxidant strategy based on optimal mitochondrial health, which has the capacity to enhance the level of hormones such as DHEA, testosterone, and the estrogens.

Taking supplements of alpha-lipoic acid; L-carnosine; classic antioxidants like vitamins A, E, C, and B_3; and active minerals and trace elements in the Krebs cycle (magnesium, selenium, zinc, and manganese) makes it possible to achieve high levels of steroid production in the mitochondria—double the organic production of hormones (an increase of 100 percent in blood values) in some 6 months of treatment![9]

In addition to renewed vitality, thanks to optimized ATP production, this nutritive, therapeutic strategy provides a physiologically normal dose of hormones, one that is adapted to the individual, with practically zero risk of cancer.

What's more, it has been speculated that what is best for internal hormone production is equally valuable for creating and restoring neurotransmitters (such as dopamine, norepinephrine, adrenaline, acetylcholine, GABA, and serotonin): as the neurons breathe better, the level of neurohormones comes back to normal, if the body is well supplied with their precursors.

5

HEALING DESTABILIZED DNA

MIRKO BELJANSKI'S ONCOTEST

In the 1970s, while conducting research at the famous Pasteur Institute on cellular DNA and the different kinds of RNA capable of regulating its activity (see chapter 2), Mirko Beljanski made another significant discovery: he observed a fundamental difference between healthy DNA and DNA in the same tissue that was becoming precancerous or even cancerous.

He found that cancerous DNA tissue always has a destabilized secondary structure compared to the DNA of healthy tissue. This destabilization

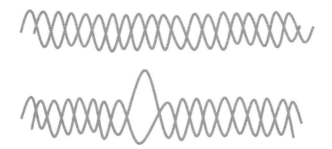

Fig. 5.1. Normal DNA (top) and destabilized DNA (bottom).

is expressed as a tendency for openings to occur between the two chains of the double helix, a tendency exacerbated by contact with everyday products, like hormones and chemical substances.

Beljanski's discovery of the difference between normal and destabilized DNA provided the foundation for him to develop a comparative test capable of determining the reactive difference between healthy DNA and cancerous DNA in the same tissue. Conducted in vitro, it measures the quantity of synthesized DNA in the presence of different known carcinogens or numerous other biological or chemical products (such as hormones and sugars).

This test—named the Oncotest—makes it possible to know in only a few minutes whether a product or a medicine will or will not have a destabilizing effect on normal and cancerous DNA, or in other words, whether the product does or does not have carcinogenic potential. In the presence of products recognized as carcinogens, healthy tissue DNA is found to be only slightly stimulated in its replication, while cancerous DNA of the same tissue is very strongly stimulated and the cell containing it divides at an accelerated rate. The result is clear: after tissue is exposed to a carcinogen in vitro, the DNA it synthesizes comprises 5 to 10 times more cancerous DNA than healthy DNA.

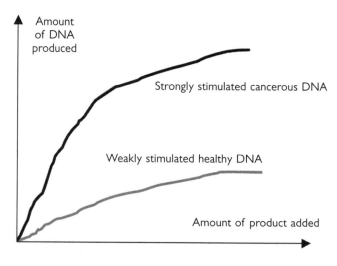

Fig. 5.2. Chart of a standard Oncotest.

This test detects the carcinogenic potential of known carcinogens and is distinct from the well-known Ames test, which confuses carcinogenesis with mutagenesis and is susceptible to false positives. The Oncotest, on the contrary, has no false positives and makes it possible to recognize the carcinogenic potential of many products that are reputedly "harmless" simply because they are not mutagenic. The Ames test does not recognize these products, even though their carcinogenic potential is expressed quite well in vivo. Among these products are numerous dyes used in cosmetics and food products, but also beta-blocking molecules and even tranquilizers used very frequently by the majority of the public.[1]

The Oncotest also makes it possible to test a number of biological substances, like hormones, and to show that they, too, have carcinogenic potential. In other words, they are DNA destabilizers *when used in non-physiological doses, particularly in their synthetic form.* This destabilization, though limited to the tissue targeted by the particular hormone, reveals the potential for hormones to induce cancer.

Thanks to recent studies on hormone replacement therapy (HRT), with close to tens of thousands of menopausal women, we know that the Oncotest's results have been verified in vivo.[2] For some forms of HRT, women in the study had a 25 percent greater chance of getting breast cancer.

But hormones are not the only substances of concern. Everyday chemical pollutants (for example, the ethylene glycol found in household products) can also destabilize the same DNA. The Oncotest is a quick tool to identify those molecules in our environment that have a lasting destabilizing effect on DNA. The three charts that follow show three Oncotests using substances with carcinogenic potential, then neutrals, and finally toxins, that is, agents that destroy the activity of the DNA polymerase used in the test.

Among substances capable of destabilizing DNA are pesticides, of which a million tons are sprayed each year into the environment. In this case as well, the Oncotest has shown the destabilizing effect of

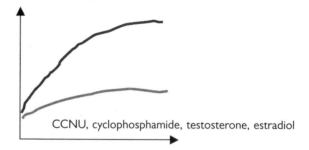

Fig. 5.3. A carcinogen slightly stimulates a healthy DNA (bottom line) and strongly stimulates an already destabilized cancerous DNA (top line).

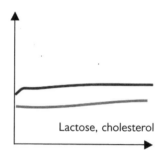

Fig. 5.4. A neutral substance affects neither healthy DNA (bottom line) nor cancerous DNA (top line).

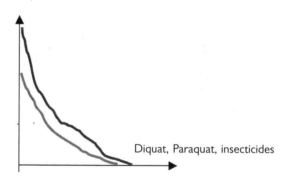

Fig. 5.5. A toxic substance inhibits the synthesis of healthy DNA (bottom line) just as much as with cancerous DNA (top line).

pesticides on DNA. In other words, it has indisputably shown their direct carcinogenic potential. Pesticides are one of the major reasons behind the increase in all types of cancers reported in the past 30 years, particularly those affecting the elimination tissues and organs (the breasts, colon, and kidneys). In France, two-thirds of waterways are polluted with more than 200 different pesticide molecules! And 5 percent of domestic sanitary installations are supplied with water that does not conform to European regulation.

It is estimated that 65 percent of the cancers found in the past 20 years could be due in part to the uncontrolled increase in these pollutants. Specifying which pollutants is unnecessary, as it is their overall effect that is most worrisome, along with the final consequence—still more damage, mutation, or even more common destabilization of cellular DNA.

Moreover, a study by the World Wildlife Fund (WWF) in the United Kingdom of 47 people (40 of whom were in Parliament) showed that close to 80 chemical pollutant substances were present in the blood of those tested, including ones, like DDT and PCB, that had been outlawed for 30 years! This means that for a very long time after exposure these chemicals remain circulating in the blood. These pollutants exert their DNA-destabilizing effect in the tissues where they are most concentrated.

The Oncotest has also indicated that a good number of chemotherapeutic substances used in high doses for fighting cancer (such as bleomycin, actinomycin, CCNU, and cyclophosphamide) are carcinogenic in lower doses. This suggests that after treatment and during the elimination phase from the body, the amount of the substance in the body is reduced and actually becomes a DNA destabilizer (that is, carcinogenic), reintroducing for a time exactly what it was supposed to eliminate!

What's worse, the various deleterious actions compound. If the same cell is subjected to excessive hormones, chemical pollution, medication, and radiation, opportunities for the DNA to increase its number of open sites increase still further. As noted in chapter 2, even those of us who are

Assimilation up to 260 nm (% increase in open sites)

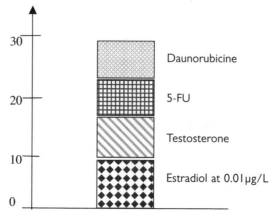

Fig. 5.6. Compounding effect of two chemotherapies
plus two hormones on DNA.

not receiving radiation treatment are exposed to an increasing amount of radiation from electromagnetic pollution, linked to the presence of cell phone relay antennas, wireless networks, computers, and telephones.

The results of these electromagnetic waves can be seen in the modification of surface proteins and also—via the calcium ion channel—in the modification of cellular membrane permeability. The effects of these alterations show up in the DNA through polyamine metabolism. Once again the DNA finds itself exposed to an increased risk of destabilization, which leads to an increased probability of the incidence of cancer, particularly leukemia and brain tumors.

At the most extreme, a DNA molecule can have 40 percent of its structure in a destabilized form, but most of the time the difference in the number of open sites between healthy DNA and destabilized DNA, or that which is becoming cancerous, is only 5 to 20 percent.

ANTI-CANCER "BOLT" MOLECULES

Mirko Beljanski's genius was evident in his decision to use the Oncotest over the course of his career as a tool to pursue further research. He presupposed that there had to be chemical substances in nature capable of acting in exactly the opposite way to carcinogens. That is to say, they would selectively inhibit the synthesis of cancerous DNA, without influencing the division of healthy DNA. These substances would appear in the Oncotest as in the following graphical representation.

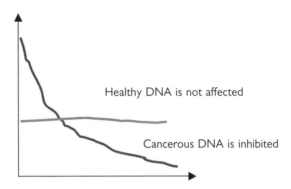

Fig. 5.7. Chart of Oncotest results with an ideal anti-cancer substance.

Mirko Beljanski discovered that, in fact, certain plant alkaloids, like alstonine from the rauwolfia plant, did have this *selective* action, capable of strongly inhibiting cancerous DNA from a number of tissues (breast, thyroid, liver, and so on), without acting on the synthesis of healthy tissue DNA. He showed that the alstonine molecule is able to penetrate the cancerous cell membrane in order to reach the destabilized DNA in the cell nucleus. Once there, the alkaloid intercalates into the purine bases of the open DNA, binding and thereby preventing the activity of enzymes that enable DNA duplication. This alkaloid does not, however, significantly penetrate healthy cells (the cellular membrane has an inverse electric charge) and does not attach to the healthy DNA.

The Oncotest makes it possible to rapidly and reproducibly test all chemical and biological substances for their potential to act selectively: with nontoxicity toward healthy tissue, while inhibiting the growth of cancerous cells. Routine use of this revolutionary test would make it possible to avoid animal experimentation in a number of circumstances. Animal experiments are as costly as they are ineffective in preventively detecting numerous harmful substances in our environment.

Spurred on by his conviction that the Oncotest would help him discover more selective anti-cancer molecules, Dr. Beljanski continued his research. He discovered that the alkaloid flavopereirine, found in another tropical plant, pao pereira from Brazil, was just as selectively anti-cancerous as alstonine in tissues with destabilized DNA (DNA contained in precancerous and cancerous cells).

The anti-cancer potential of these two alkaloids, alstonine and flavopereirine, has been verified in numerous animal, plant, and human cancer tissues (17 different cell lines), as well as on human DNA isolated following surgical excision.

The charts of results below show that the two products do not affect the growth of healthy tissues cultured in vitro.

The rauwolfia alkaloid of alstonine first studied by Mirko Beljanski showed better activity in hormonally dependent tissues. Moreover, its specifically anti-cancer effect also seemed to bring about hormonal regulation so effectively that it was recommended to menopausal women

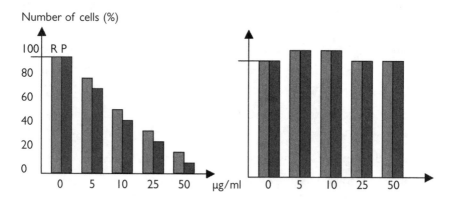

Fig. 5.8. The inhibition of G-361 melanoma cells by pao pereira (P) and Rauwolfia vomitoria (R) extracts on the left. On the right, the absence of the same inhibiting action when using pao pereira and rauwolfia extracts on a line of healthy cells, fibroblasts CCD-974Sk.

for treating symptoms like hot flashes, and to men and young women for combating certain types of infertility.

The alkaloid discovered and extracted from pao pereira, flavopereirine, a molecule even smaller than alstonine, showed, in addition to its anti-cancer effects, a strong antiviral potential, effective on plant viruses (tobacco mosaic virus), animal viruses (cat FIV, dog influenza), and human viruses (hepatitis C, influenza, HIV).

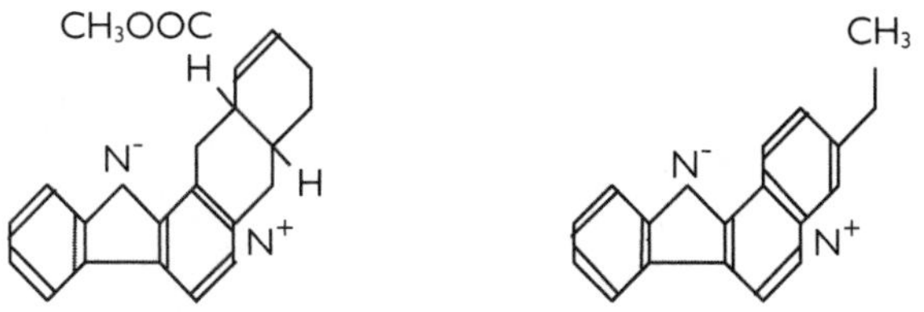

Fig. 5.9. Two anti-cancer alkaloids.

These two products, which are active against in vitro cancer DNA, have been shown to improve chances of recovery in some cancer patients. Flavopereirine is effective in vivo even within the central nervous system, since, because of its small size, it can traverse the blood-brain barrier.

After more than 40 years of research Mirko Beljanski thus demonstrated that natural substances from specific plant extracts were able to selectively control the destabilization of DNA in vivo, even within the brain. He nicknamed his two alkaloids "bolt" molecules because they were capable of filling open DNA sites and blocking them if the destabilized DNA belonged to precancerous or cancerous cells. Because the duplication of DNA is vital to the existence of a cell, when duplication is prevented, the cell dies.

Since DNA is able to repair itself less effectively as it ages, it tends toward progressive, continuing destabilization and even chromosomal breakage. Over time, if the cell with destabilized DNA does not die,

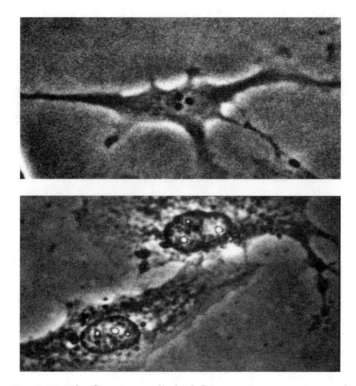

Fig. 5.10. The fluorescent alkaloid flavopereirine remains on the outside·of the healthy cell (top) but penetrates the nucleus and the nucleoli of the cancerous cell (bottom).

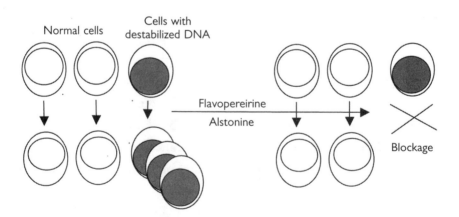

Fig. 5.11. Normal cells (left) are contrasted with cells with destabilized DNA (center). "Bolt" molecules make it possible to prevent these harmful DNA from duplicating (right).

there is a high risk of unregulated division and, ultimately, cancer development. It is thus very important to have molecules at our disposal—like we have today in pao pereira and rauwolfia extracts—with the potential for blocking replication of destabilized DNA before it degenerates into actual cancer.

ANTI-AGING SYNERGY OF THE TWO ALKALOIDS

Faced with the very troubling health threat of various pollutants in our environment, it is certainly comforting to be able to have at our disposal "bolt" molecules, which are potentially capable of eliminating cells whose DNA has been either damaged by environmental toxins or destabilized following chronic exposure to extremely low-frequency radiation.

Pao pereira and rauwolfia alkaloids also appear to modulate the production of hormones that control the endocrine glands. With age, cerebral hormone synthesis decreases, while the somatic glands become less sensitive to these hormones. Blocking aberrant DNA in the brain and at the epithelium core makes it possible to normalize the active hormone-receptor cell pair.

Substances such as the pao pereira and rauwolfia extracts are thus invaluable in the realm of anti-aging strategies, in several ways.

- They can be used to preventively block cells with destabilized DNA—whatever the cause—before they form actual tumors.
- These two natural extracts, which penetrate only cells with destabilized DNA, will also attach to mitochondrial DNA, which is responsible for the synthesis of enzymes helpful to respiration. These cells, on the path to their own demise, will be removed from circulation all the more quickly.
- They may also affect the cellular nuclei in bodily tissues, making it possible, particularly for the endocrine glands, to regularize hormone

production. If, after controlling for blood and other deficiencies, hormones (such as thyroid hormones, steroids, or others) are prescribed on account of the effects of age, these plant extracts represent a possible safeguard against future DNA destabilization in the tissues targeted by the prescribed hormones.

- As we have seen, the flavopereirine molecule is small enough to penetrate the blood-brain barrier, and it will enter only cells with DNA on its way to degeneration or dedifferentiation. So it may actually be able to reconstruct the brain's "hard disk drive."

- The flavopereirine alkaloid, which attaches to purine bases in open DNA, also attaches to purine bases in RNA and DNA viruses and deactivates them.

- The flavopereirine molecule is of even greater interest due to its demonstrated regulating/inhibiting effect on a cell's overproduction of interleukin-6—a cytokine that is inflammatory and inhibits stem cell reconstruction, particularly of neuronal stem cells.[3] As we have seen, chronic tissue inflammation is a troubling characteristic of premature aging that can be fought only by precise, selective nutritive measures (see chapter 1) as well as by a synergy of actions to improve cellular aerobic respiration (see chapter 3). As the cells begin to "unclog" themselves, to use Dr. Seignalet's words,[4] pao pereira extract can be used in conjunction with omega-3 fatty acids in order to nourish the membranes and synapses and to suppress the inflammatory response induced by interleukin-6.

- An even more powerful combination of strategies is one founded on the use of RNA fragments. Stimulating the DNA in the bone marrow with an RNA primer makes it possible to modulate an immune system that is perhaps failing locally, and to harness the reparative power of stem cells to act as micro-surgeons on tissues developing fibrosis or degenerating.

These powerful effects are the basis for the following anti-aging recommendations:

- Take the pao pereira extract 2 times a month, 3 times a year, in order to protect cellular DNA, particularly neuronal DNA.
- Take preventive treatments of rauwolfia extracts 2 or 3 times a year to support the capacity of your tissues to renew themselves without functional loss or dedifferentiation.
- Consider reinforcing the capacity for stem cell repair by taking RNA fragments.

CASE STUDIES

Bolt Molecules, Ginkgo, and RNA Fragments

Louise M.'s case is an extreme example showing RNA fragment stimulation of bone marrow stem cells over the course of a chemotherapy known to be toxic to bone marrow. It also demonstrates the use of bolt molecules to act in conjunction with anti-cancer drugs to prevent development of cancer.

Louise M., born in 1954, was a smoker for 30 years before she quit in 2003. Unfortunately, she was diagnosed with small cell lung cancer in March 2004, with many metastases along the lymph node mediastinal chain, as well as in the liver and the adrenal glands.

The prognosis was considered to be hopeless; physicians predicted maximum survival time of 6 months with medial treatment. Despite this, chemotherapy treatment was started anyway. Each session lasted 3 to 4 days and involved a combination of epirubicin, carboplatin, and cisplatin. In total, there were 6 sessions conducted every 3 weeks from April to August 2004.

An additional protocol was proposed by her treating physician that was based on "bolt" molecules of pao pereira and rauwolfia extracts (for synergy of action with alkylating chemotherapy and targeted DNA), along with ginkgo extracts and RNA fragments in order to restore the level of leukocytes and platelets, which can be dramatically lowered, particularly with epirubicin. A cellular nutritherapy strategy of fish-based fatty acids, antioxidants, and high doses of probiotics was concurrently begun.

It is important to note that the patient's levels of red blood cells, leukocytes, and platelets stayed in the same normal range despite large initial fluctuations following chemotherapy drips. Her overall immunity at the end of chemotherapy remained good, which, for the patient, represented a real chance to prevent her cancer from recurring.

Following 6 chemotherapy sessions, the doctors warned Louise that her brain, relatively unaffected by the drugs used, would have to be treated with radiation therapy with 15 sessions in total, in order to best prevent an eventual cerebral metastasis. Radiation is invaluable for destroying a tumor, but in order to do so it produces a lot of free radicals. Complete, diffuse radiation of the brain is, therefore, an extremely destructive treatment, inducing accelerated aging in the site affected.

The patient underwent these sessions while continuing to take RNA fragments, anti-fibrosis ginkgo and pao pereira in order to block DNA on the path to destabilizing. During the sessions, she also took 800 mg/day of SAMe in order to maximize cerebral protection. On the recommendation of her doctor, Louise has continued to take these products as part of the "biological method." They allowed her to undergo further treatment without the damage to healthy cells caused by the aggressiveness of conventional therapies.

Contrary to the prognosis of her oncologists, the patient enjoyed complete remission of her original cancer and various metastases. Her general condition has become, in her opinion and those of her friends, better than ever! (See the chart on page 83.)

Bolt Molecules and Hormonal Regulation

Susie R. was born in 1929. From the age of 39, she suffered from panic attacks, leaving her completely dependent and distressed. Twenty years later, her attacks led to anorexia and depression. Her treating physician, following a blood test, detected Hashimoto's disease with an extremely elevated level of anti-thyroid antibodies.

The only treatment offered was thyroid extracts, which did not

TABLE 5.1. THE CASE OF LOUISE M.

Blood Formula Count	Date Analyzed	Red Blood Cells millions/mm³	Hemoglobin	Hematocrit	Leukocytes thousands/mm³	Neutrophils %	Lymphocytes %	Monocytes %	Platelets X 1000
1st chemo on April 10-15	04/23 04/30 05/07	3.91 3.59 3.59	11.8 11.0 10.9	34.6 31.5 31.5	10.8 05.3 13.9	53.7 16.2 40.0	41.7 70.4 57.0	1.8 9.9 2.0	311 234 764
2nd chemo on May 10-13	05/17 05/24 05/28	3.61 3.36 3.28	10.7 10.1 10.1	31.4 28.4 29.4	10.9 09.1 06.7	59.6 38.6 17.0	37.3 50.6 75.0	2.0 9.2 2.0	476 217 260
3rd chemo on June 1-4	06/07 06/14 06/21 06/25	3.67 3.22 3.73 4.07	11.7 10.4 12.0 13.0	34.1 29.9 35.8 39.0	08.9 06.1 04.9 08.0	54.0 28.3 21.0 37.0	40.9 63.8 76.0 61.0	2.6 6.4 1.0 0.0	624 192 427 657
4th chemo on June 28-30	07/05 07/12 07/16	4.07 3.94 4.10	13.0 12.9 14.0	39.0 38.4 41.0	08.0 07.7 03.7	37.0 55.6 38.0	61.0 40.8 54.0	0.0 2.1 2.0	617 415 152
5th chemo on July 20-22	07/23 07/29 08/05 08/09	4.32 3.99 4.40 4.35	14.0 13.5 15.5 15.5	43.0 40.0 45.0 44.0	11.5 06.4 03.1 06.0	79.0 50.9 23.0 51.0	12.9 42.6 68.0 45.0	6.1 5.0 6.0 4.0	463 386 091 216
6th chemo on August 10-12	08/18 08/25 09/01 09/08	4.08 4.19 4.28 4.34	13 14 14 14	40 42 43 44	04.2 03.6 06.5 09.4	54.6 13.0 40.0 49.6	40.8 86.0 55.0 41.4	3.0 1.0 4.0 7.0	335 062 356 443
After the chemo-therapies	09/15 09/22	4.35 4.97	14 14	43 42	06.9 07.4	48.9 53.6	39.7 34.7	9.0 8.4	275 185

In spite of 6 intensive chemotherapy sessions, the rate of leukocytes and platelets stayed at a quasi-normal level; thanks to this conserved or even improved immunity, a reasonable hope exists that we could see a lasting remission of the cancer in the future.

ultimately help offset the gland's underproduction. Instead they led to weight gain, digestive problems, and the persistent feeling that her body was frozen, all of which caused great emotional distress. Enzyme treatment assays and calcium EAP injections helped her for a time, but her condition ultimately worsened.

On the advice of a friend, she went to a therapist who prescribed her 4 pao pereira gel caps per day as well as 4 ginkgo gel caps and 1 dose of RNA fragments per week. At the end of 3 months, all of the troubles from which she had been suffering had disappeared: her digestion was better, her skin pigments returned to normal, and her general condition was good. She has since continued to take the products to maximize the functioning of her underproductive thyroid and allow her to lead a normal life.

Menopause-Related Problems

Nicole M. was born in 1944. Ever since childhood, she had worked in farming. At the age of 56, she experienced the first symptoms of menopause, with extreme hot flashes, intermittent insomnia, weight gain, and problems related to vaginal dryness.

She refused the hormone replacement therapy suggested by her doctor because of some alarming information she had read regarding such treatments. She thus went without treatment for 2 years and began to suffer from pain in the back and bones. A bone density examination revealed advanced osteoporosis, particularly along the spinal cord.

On the advice of a friend, she consulted a doctor who advised her to take 2 gel caps of rauwolfia a day. The results were immediate. Her hot flashes disappeared and the punishing pain she experienced in her bones diminished noticeably. She followed this supplementation regimen for 12 months, followed by a break of 3 to 6 months. During this time, she once again began to experience bone pain, whereupon she again began to take 2 gel caps per day, which allowed her to lead a normal life.

Alstonine therefore appears to be a good means of regulating hormonal problems that may develop at the onset of menopause. Taking amino acid supplements (glycine, arginine, glutamine), somatotropin precursors, in silicon and in iodine, and SAMe could help menopausal women's conditions even more.

6

THE HEALTH HOLOGRAM

A hologram could be described as a three-dimensional photograph, an image of an object made by a laser and recorded on a special holographic plate (see the appendix, "Holography and Holograms," for further explanation). One of the most remarkable features of a hologram is that even a small part of it—when illumined by the light of the same laser—will recreate the entire original image. In this way it is unlike a typical photographic negative, pieces of which will reflect only their particular part of the whole. Thus, a hologram can be seen as a mosaic in which each piece reflects the whole from a particular angle.

If the body is seen as a hologram, four major functions, and only four, are found at the macro- and microscopic level. In terms of prevention, which is fundamental to any anti-aging program, or in terms of therapy, during and after a specific intervention, it is necessary to once again establish an optimal interaction among bodily functions.

The hologram model can also be used to represent the way in which our individual health is maintained by an ensemble of dietary, hygienic, and supplementary measures, all working for the same purpose: optimizing cellular function. We can graph this ensemble of measures in a rectangle containing all of the methods to present an instant summary of what works for each one of us for optimal longevity.

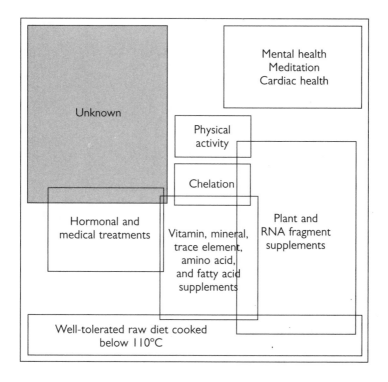

Fig. 6.1. Hologram of a health program.

- A part of this rectangle remains unknown: it represents what we do not yet know in terms of care and prevention but, once known, will allow us to better care for ourselves in the future. We expect this will include cellular therapy using stem cells or even biophysics, as well as the whole of what biochemistry can already offer us.

- The base of this rectangle is good macronutrition, because it is unthinkable to ignore or to neglect what we ingest every day if we hope to construct a valuable anti-aging plan: this daily intake completely renews our cellular makeup almost every seven years! Externally it remains identical, but the internal matter renews itself completely based on what we eat.

- Micronutrition—the essential intake of vitamins, minerals, trace elements, and fatty acids—is shown in another rectangle, partially superimposed on the first, because these two aspects are interrelated.

- Also included in this hologram are natural extracts, coming primarily from plants, such as those described in this book, source of the molecules such as alstonine and flavopereirine that favorably impact DNA.
- In our modern and polluted world, chelation of heavy metals takes priority, so it is placed at the heart of these prevention measures.
- Physical exercise, meditation techniques, and mental health management are part of a comprehensive strategy for well-being and cellular vitality.
- The health hologram also includes medical treatments, which also implies hormonal supplements, because people who are 50 or older have rarely reached that age without the help of one or two medicines or hormones taken regularly—all products that continuously support their vitality.

CONSTRUCTING YOUR HEALTH HOLOGRAM

In concrete terms, most people over 40, faced with fatigue, stress, and the passing of time (!), realize that they are losing their vitality. Initially they may look for a few small ways to modify this loss of mental and physical performance. At first, vitamins may provide positive changes, but they are only temporarily masking the true causes of chronic fatigue.

However, the information presented in this book will help you—ideally with the help of a health professional—to build your own personalized program. Guided by the suggestions provided and coordinated with the model of the hologram, you can construct a health program that will be both comprehensive and adapted to you, which will help ensure its effectiveness.

Your health hologram will comprise several facets of varying

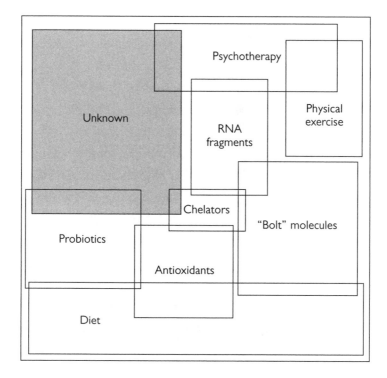

Fig. 6.2. You are unique and should individualize the general model to create your health program hologram.

importance. It will differ depending on whether you do or do not suffer from chronic digestive problems, whether or not you are physically active on a regular basis, and whether you show signs of obesity or, to the contrary, of being underweight. Your anti-aging program will also differ in intensity, depending on whether you are starting at 45 or at 75.

In sum, this unique program is dictated by your individual medical history and the urgency behind attaining certain objectives (weight, vitality, state of mucous membranes/skin, hormonal balance). These factors will guide the importance accorded to each of the hologram's elements. The hologram is also contingent on your ability to fully follow the program, the parameter that is the most difficult for a doctor or advising biologist to manage. You, along with your treating therapist, must take the lead in creating the foundation for a healthy future . . . in order to make the most of your body over the course of time, and to maximize your health.

A Comprehensive Strategy, Not a Product

The model of the hologram, suggesting a three-dimensional image and multiple sides of an object, subject, or, in this case, health program, makes it possible to immediately realize that the issue at hand must be approached from many angles. The more comprehensive the strategy, the more scientific and the more successful it will be. This principle is the same whether you are focusing on prevention or the treatment of degeneration that has already begun. The only difference in the overall program would be reflected in dosage and intensity.

A comprehensive, individualized strategy that concerns all parts of the body—guaranteed by the use of a health hologram—rather than one based on a few products makes it possible to enhance the work of therapists and patients using techniques for prevention and optimized health.

Of course, the products mentioned in this book are precious tools, and there is no shortage of examples showing that their effects are powerful, beneficial, and often the determining factor in improvement. But they must be part of a comprehensive plan to be successful. A biological product, even though very valuable, can act effectively only if the cells that receive it are functioning well and have optimized respiration, if the acidity of the cytoplasm is in a normal range, and if the catalysts are there. This "groundwork" is an indispensable precondition.

Mirko Beljanski, whose work has been cited several times in this book, understood that in order to be accepted by the body, such products must be as close as possible to living substances; in other words, they must be truly biological, whether they are vitamins, hormones, coenzymes, or plant extracts. He surrounded himself with a team of doctors and biologists who were able, on a better level than he, to gauge the physiological effect of the various substances he was researching.

He observed, for example, that his biological products had to be administered concurrently with catalysts like magnesium or zinc, without which the effectiveness of the product would be compromised. The alkaloids, which normally situate themselves in the DNA molecule, must not be inhibited or destroyed while en route to their targets. The cytoplasm's pH level, the quantity of intracellular calcium, the cellular membrane's potential, and so on—regulation of all these factors is important in order to get the most from a product. Many of these parameters (such as the cytoplasmic pH and the level of intracellular calcium) are predicated upon good cellular aerobics, which leads to the production of ATP and a number of movements of molecules and minerals between the cell and its surrounding area. And when the Krebs cycle is partially inhibited, nothing else takes place and even the best products will be only partially effective.

Clearly, the research conducted by Professor Mirko Beljanski from 1950 to 1998 belongs to the twenty-first century in its visionary and comprehensive—holographic—view of biological phenomena. We thus hope that this book will contribute to making his pioneering work known and to widening its scope of application.

A COMPREHENSIVE ANTI-AGING PROGRAM

The goal of this book is for each person to become familiar with, and later implement, simple strategies for use—at the level both of the cell and of the body as a whole—in order to best face and benefit from the passing of time. Understanding the body itself as a hologram, whose multiple facets are the cells, ensures that we do not forget the measures to take on the macroscopic level, nor the important ones on the microscopic level.

Anti-Aging Program for the Cells
As we have seen, the fact that the body is composed of tissues originating from three original embryonic layers, themselves responsible for

four principal functions, provides a basic understanding of the healthy functioning of our cells.

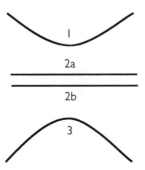

Fig. 6.3. As we know, the body has three fundamental tissues and four functions.

The program on the microscopic level can be summarized as follows:

- Nutrition necessary for each cell, regardless of the specific tissue in question:
  - ▸ Purified water with mild mineral content and somewhat acidic pH (preferably nonoxidized, with an average oxido-reduction potential between 23 and 25)
  - ▸ A good quantity of high-quality protein (0.36 g per pound of weight per day)
  - ▸ Sugar conforming to daily expenditure of energy and no more
  - ▸ Omega-3 and omega-6 fatty acids, with an ideal ratio of 1 to 5 respectively
  - ▸ Natural vitamins A, C, E, D, and B complex; minerals (calcium, magnesium, and potassium, along with monitoring of iron levels to assure neither excess nor deficiency); trace elements (zinc, selenium, manganese, boron, and chromium); and first-degree antioxidants

- Specific supplementary protocol for external protection, assimilation, and elimination provided by the mucous membranes (endoderm):
  ‣ Tests for food intolerances (based on IgE/IgG) should be run as soon as signs of chronic intestinal or inflammatory troubles are seen (the same as in the case of obesity).
  ‣ Probiotics should be taken as needed to aid digestion and repair the intestinal mucous membrane. Probiotics are also the essential element in localized immune tolerance.
  ‣ L-glutamine—the fuel for permanent renewal of intestinal cells—should be supplemented as needed.

- Specific supplementary protocol for internal structure and defense (mesoderm):
  ‣ RNA fragments are the most precise stimulants for cells of the immune system, while at the same time being bone marrow stem cell replicators, capable of repairing all the tissues.

- Specific supplementary protocol for the creation and circulation of energy (mesoderm):
  ‣ Acetyl-L-carnitine, which facilitates the transport of fatty acids in the mitochondria
  ‣ Alpha-lipoic acid, powerful anti-radical and first-degree antioxidant regenerator
  ‣ S-adenosyl-methionine (SAMe), detoxification and reconstruction agent
  ‣ Natural heavy metal chelators (garlic, coriander, chlorella, selenium, and so on)
  ‣ *Ginkgo biloba* extract from the tree's golden leaves, for its anti-fibrosis and regulatory action

- Specific supplementary protocol for memory and coordination:
  ‣ The intake of amino acids, precursors to the growth hormone, or neurotransmitters

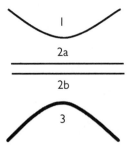

Fig. 6.4. Probiotics and tests for food intolerances for the mucous membrane lining.

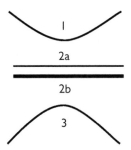

Fig. 6.5. RNA fragments for immunity.

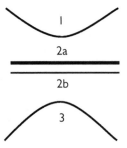

Fig. 6.6. Second-degree antioxidants, chelators, and ginkgo for energy production.

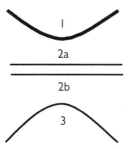

*Fig. 6.7. Hormones, amino acids, specific nutrients, and
"bolt" molecules for the brain and for the DNA of destabilized cells.*

▸ The intake of particular fractions of lipids, like phosphatidylserine and lecithin extracts

▸ Supplementation and protection using "bolt" molecules (alstonine, flavopereirine) in order to eliminate destabilized cells that
are degenerating or potentially cancerous

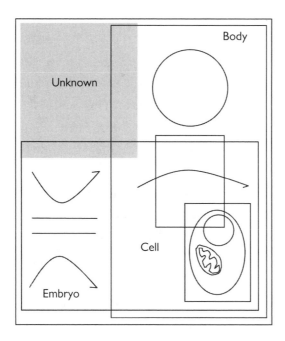

*Fig. 6.8. This hologram reflects the embryo, the adult body,
and the cell, all based on identical functions.*

► Supplementation of deficient hormones (such as progesterone, testosterone, and DHEA) and peptides (such as HGH, melatonin, thyroid, and thymic peptides) presents certain risks. Supplementation is a choice that can be made only with the help of an informed therapist, as taking supplements is not without the risk of destabilizing DNA in the targeted tissues. If hormone therapy becomes necessary, it is an especially good idea to also take the "bolt" molecules.

Anti-Aging Program for the Whole Body

Since the body is itself a hologram, whose multiple facets are the cells in each tissue, the supplements contributing to each part will, of course, reinforce the whole structure. Likewise, the following simple, good-sense measures complement those just listed; they are valuable in terms of overall well-being and indirectly reinforce cell vitality.

• A healthy diet, founded on fresh, organic, living, unprocessed foods, raw or steamed.

• A moderate, regular dose of physical exercise (such as walking, biking, gymnastics, and so on), included in the workday if possible, especially for people under stress. This can be beneficially augmented with the practice of cardiac coherence and practices such as yoga, qi gong, and tai chi, which integrate body movements with breathing exercises.

• Mental or spiritual activities (such as reading, meditation, benevolent activity, social meetings, and so on) are indispensable for every human being, both for enriching our own experience and memory and also for meeting other human beings and literally being enriched by their lives.

A complete human being thus needs selected foods, energy, and spirituality to be fully enriched, to live, and to go through time with a minimum of damage. Most importantly, the measures detailed in chapters 1 through 5 and summarized here are interdependent yet also synergistic.

With the passage of time, it does not help to play games with your body or abuse it by following the latest fads in diet or supplements for short periods of time. Simply put, to live well, remember that the body, both microcosmically and macrocosmically, can be described as having four functions, which give rise to four needs: protecting the body's borders, reinforcing its internal structure and defense, increasing its capacity for energy production, and preserving memory and coordination. *This is the comprehensive anti-aging regimen!*

Appendix

HOLOGRAPHY AND HOLOGRAMS

The words *holistic* and *holographic* have nowadays become quite popular, appearing in newspapers and in many recent books.

The primary use of the term *holography* describes the recording of data onto a medium, as is done in photography or computer programming. However, it can also refer to a model that can be figuratively applied to a subject in order to better understand a problem, whether it be medical, biological, philosophical, or spiritual.

In biology, the most famous defender of the holographic model to this day is K. H. Pribram,[1] who has been defending this model since 1974—already 30 years! This professor of neurophysiology was essentially the first to come out with the hypothesis that the brain functions like a holographic model and that images in memory are in fact virtual holographic images, naturally and continuously reconstituted by different sites in the cortex.

How is this conceivable, and what does the word *hologram* mean in everyday life? By definition, a hologram is a three-dimensional (3-D) image of an object, obtained through the interference between a referential laser and the light reflected by the same laser source off the object being holographed. The impression of the image is made on a plate produced with a thick resin.

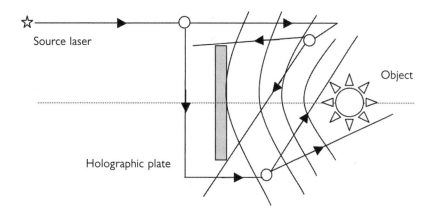

Fig. A.1. Creation of a hologram.

Once a hologram is recorded onto the holographic plate, one can easily see the 3-D image of the object by exposing the plate to the same laser used during the image's recording.

Depending on the position of the observer and the light source with respect to the plate during reconstruction, the 3-D image appears in front or behind the illuminated plate; the image looks real or, rather, virtual.

A hologram has two important features:

• Several images can be superimposed on the same plate, using a different laser source for each.

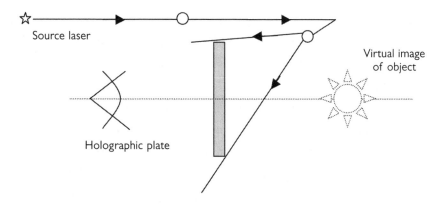

Fig. A.2. Recreation of a hologram.

- If one were to break the plate with the image recorded on it into five or ten pieces, one would get five or ten full images of the object, more or less distorted, but still whole.

The sum of all these related images, seen at a certain angle from the object, gives the most fair, precise, and comprehensive 3-D image.

Each part, however, remains representative of the whole.

Since its invention by British professor Dennis Gabor in 1960, who received the Nobel Prize at the time for his work, the holographic technique has found multiple applications.

In the industrial world this technique is used primarily to represent a 3-D object as precisely as possible. This has allowed professionals to predict sections, cut within $^1/_{100}$ mm, in an object to be manufactured.

In biology, researchers in neuropsychology, following K. H. Pribram, have used this hologram model to explain the recreation of images by the brain during the memorization process.

It is thus possible to draw an analogy between the image recorded onto a plate and the sum of images recorded in the cortex, which acts like a living holographic plate in a constant state of change. Synapses, or the membrane intersections between neurons, are most likely the place where the holographic film of our lives is recorded. The cortex can thus record, by superimposing them in the same area, an infinite number of photos and films over the length of a lifetime, which will be re-created depending on the particular "lighting" and in particular circumstances (analogous to the different lasers used in the creation of the hologram).

Each re-created, that is, remembered, image is, in effect, the compilation of several pieces of information disseminated in several different geographic areas of the cortex (right, left, front, back, lateral, and so on) The best overall memory thus comes from superimposing all these data.

The reconstituted mental image is really *virtual,* because it does not exist anywhere but in the confluence of all the cortical zones. It

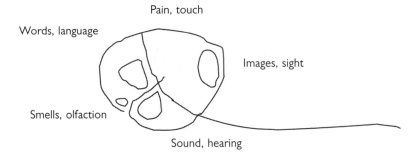

Fig. A.3. Remembered effects converge in the cortex.

is created thanks to a stimulus, like light, a sound, or an image, by which one accesses a picture vaster than anything known before. It is the memory that emerges.

For example, you are looking at a photo of your grandmother. Then you remember the party during which the photo was taken. Your uncle and your three nephews were there and made a lot of noise, which had angered you. Your mother had baked a huge cake that you can still smell and taste. An orchestra played wonderful music that a friend was able to record for you at the time.

The smells, music, images, and associated emotions are all a part of the same picture, unique and coherent. In order to reconstitute it, you have to call upon stored information from different areas, each trace of memory awaking another, for an increasingly accurate overall view.

This image is a beautiful hologram, such as one makes every day, pratically every second of one's life. Creating connections between images requires a medium, that is to say, the cerebral cortex.

Doctors have recently rediscovered this everyday reality by developing a reanimation technique that is both simple and quite practical.

At Garches Hospital in France, not far from Paris, there is a clinic for those with severe trauma who have just come out of deep and prolonged comas. Upon waking, they are offered a chance to reeducate their memory using a palette of scents.

Therapists in this somewhat unusual clinic primarily ask questions about the family and olfactory preferences of the patient. If a relative reminds them of the scent of strawberries or chocolate, or something the person used to enjoy in particular, the designated scent is tested by presenting it to the patient.

Usually, at the time of their admission, people suffering from trauma can neither move nor speak, but these scents awaken in them past emotions that they associated with the same words that they now are having trouble pronouncing. And it works! With patience, thanks to a familiar scent, the people whose brains underwent a terrible shock slowly but surely regain their memory, including images, words, sensations, and emotions.

Why use scent memory? Perhaps because the olfactory passages are the only ones that take care to avoid the *thalamus,* that huge sensory sorting station, which can be an obstacle in itself, as it is sometimes the site of lesions that remain unrepaired, before rejoining the cortex, the paleocortex, or the rhinencephalis.

Thanks to this method for facilitating access to the cortex (a method that is both rapid and unrestricted), the first aspect of memory, the olfactory sense, can be accessed. This stimulus leads to other cerebral areas, where other types of information are stored. Combined with

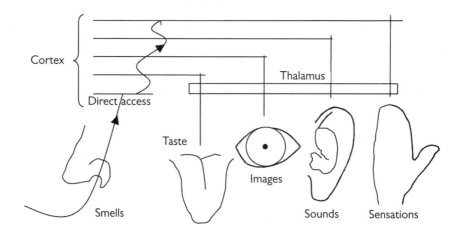

Fig. A.4. The cortex resembles a holographic plate.

the desire to reconstitute the image, even with a few mistakes, it is possible to create a coherent virtual holographic image of the item smelled and to elicit the word attributed to it.

The cortex is thus very much a holographic plate that can be illuminated with a single type of light; it reconstitutes little by little all informative content in order to re-create the rounded-out image of a memory.

Figuratively, it makes sense to use this model of a hologram in order to understand different objects, different subjects, and, more generally, *different realities* that we are considering.

Holography is part of our physiology, and observing everything with the aid of this multifaceted prism should be, theoretically and practically, the most accurate and comprehensive method possible.

Thus in modern life, if a woman observes a man, she will first perceive a silhouette, then hear his voice, and finally catch his eye. This already gives her three different types of information on the same subject. She will then learn who he is, what he does, and how he behaves toward others—all the aspects of his personality. She will perhaps listen to the opinions others have of him. She will learn about his interests, his dislikes, his habits . . . in fact, she is going to create the most comprehensive hologram of this man, one that will give her the most information and make it possible for her to optimize any communication with him.

This way of doing things is natural. Nothing is more common than this system employed by the mind. As soon as we wish to be exact, we produce the largest holograms possible in order to have the most intimate knowledge of a subject or observed object.

This model of the hologram can also be referred to when describing what occurs to our memory when we listen to someone speak in a foreign language. We might be familiar with a certain number of words in Spanish but still find it nearly impossible to completely follow the very rapid speech of a native Spanish speaker. Several holes in comprehension appear. Our brain tries to reconstitute little by little the sentences and ideas of the speaker, but this still is sometimes very vague. If too much of the speech remains an unknown it approaches nonsense, which is sometimes the source of much hilarity! The brain calls on partial memory and, thanks to an assembly of already known references, ends up reconstructing an image faithful to the thought of the speaker, almost as if we were able to erase the blanks and reconstruct the speaker's exact thought: partial memory, but yet a message that is almost perfectly reconstructed.

On the cellular level, it has recently been shown that DNA—the cell's version of the brain—functions in much the same way. In order to treat myopathy, a genetic illness in which muscle proteins are not correctly synthesized, researchers have been practicing "axon skipping": they mask the defective gene using a small piece of RNA that stops the continuous irritation that was causing the continuously faulty protein synthesis.

Better to have silence than send the wrong message! DNA will thus produce usable protein once again, slightly truncated perhaps (partial memory), but functional.

If DNA, in order to produce proteins, is also creating a "hologram" by drawing on the genes in different areas of memory that it needs, and if in so doing it reconstructs each message that is good and useful to it, then the analogy with cerebral memory is faithful overall.

The consequences are huge, since this means that genetic memory is everywhere and nowhere all at once, just like cerebral memory! It means that the more complex the organism, the richer the memory and, thus, the more locations in which memory is stored, even when we are talking about standard proteins basic to cellular life. It is the combination of several genes (several pieces of memory, sometimes with one or two blanks) that makes a good protein, but that we've known for a long time!

But what's the value of the American research project that, for $1.3 billion, had hoped to identify the famous cancer genes in hopes of offering a cancer treatment? If DNA is a hologram, one can already see that this project will be useless. Cancer genes will always be somewhere other than the place from which sites implicated in controlling cancer have been driven out. Memory does not exist in a fixed location, since the virtual image reconstituted for protein production stems from several locations and is the result of an interaction or interference among several transmitter sites.

In the same way that cerebral memory is stored in multiple locations, with the necessary relays for its arrival at the cortex, genetic memory will also be the result of several active and inactive sites. It will be (is) an image, a momentary interaction and not an object . . .

This simple reflection on holograms and the analogies it offers between two types of memory should make it possible for "scientists" (and especially those who finance them) to avoid costly research mistakes.

As you can see, this small book's value, dear reader who has had the

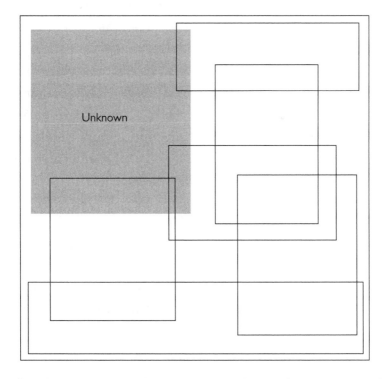

Fig. A.5. A person's complete hologram can be visualized as a rectangle containing all gathered data. A part of this hologram is unknown as much for the doctor as for the patient himself.

patience to keep reading up until this point, is tremendous, a savings of no less than $1.3 billion for the American people if just one enlightened official should get to this page.

Besides, wanting to treat cancer patients with gene therapy is clearly the idea of a geneticist who has never consulted a sick patient in his life, a researcher who is woefully incomplete in his approach that is, thus, nonscientific. Cancer merits more than anything else a multifaceted approach, a hologram-like vision, in which the largest variety of medical and paramedical disciplines would be integrated.

Thus, if a doctor sees a patient during a consultation, he must know what he eats and drinks, where he lives, when the symptoms first appeared, whether he has family problems. He quizzes him about his work and habits. He then calls on a number of blood and urine tests; if needed, radiographs, echography, an MRI, and other tests are ordered. All these questions and techniques make it possible for the doctor to construct a multifaceted hologram of his patient.

In matters of treatment, it should also logically be necessary to look to a therapeutic hologram in order to reestablish biological equilibrium. The more difficult and complex a problem, the more one should consider all possible methods of reasoning in order to bring the patient the most comprehensive, and thus the most effective, solutions according to holographic logic and according to logic in general.

Not all solutions have the same significance.

In the case of serious septicemia, the equation (bacteria = illness) is accurate almost 100 percent of the time; you have to act quickly and effectively in injecting antibiotics, as they represent the patient's best chance for survival. After this first treatment, the body can come to restabilize on its own and make it so that the bacteria no longer develops.

For cancer, on the other hand, the causes are numerous and complex: the equation (cancer = tumor) is not accurate because it is incomplete, so much so that if you remove the tumor without worrying about the quantity of polyamines in the intestine, the health of the bone marrow,

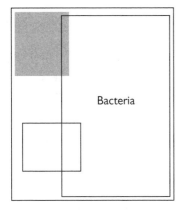 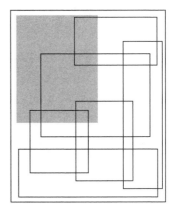

Bacteria

Fig. A.6. Left: Septicemia. Quite well known. Treatable by antibiotics. Right: Cancer, which has several unknowns, various causes, and complementary therapies.

the status of aerobic cellular respiration, hormonal balance in the most general sense, viral and/or vaccination history, mental health, or even the amplitude of the patient's personal magnetic field, there is a high probability of relapse.

Comprehensive research is a necessity, especially for all these patients who do not have time on their hands: one must act quickly and correctly, not only according to protocol imposed by a popular product or cocktail of products, but according to holographic logic, which aims to optimally reestablish the four bodily functions. It is simple and safe.

Taking away a localized tumor, even by sophisticated means (selective chemotherapy, radio-immunology), and then contenting oneself with regular checkups using increasingly refined medical imaging is, holographically, unwise because it is not comprehensive. Nothing has been done to change the conditions that caused the problem, leaving them to possibly cause a future relapse.

In such a case the treating therapist's instinct was not wrong but incomplete. Thus patients leaving the hospital after a cancer-related operation often seek out alternative or complementary medicines. They know quite well that their treatment has not taken into account their whole self to ensure their future recovery. They also know that they have to take this step quickly. Depending on the stage of advancement of the disease and the willingness of the patient, it is important to activate certain elements, such as those described in this book. Ten opinions are worth more than one or two. How many are implemented is limited only by the patient himself—by what he can accept, follow, and understand.

The hologram model makes it possible to construct the ideal program for a person, not leaving out any important aspects, with regard to the four major functions described in the preceding pages; for a doctor, to train in the holographic or holistic method is to expand one's training rather than to make it more specialized.

Specialists are vital to technical disciplines, like reanimation, imagery, surgery, and osteopathy (without exclusion). Nonspecialists or

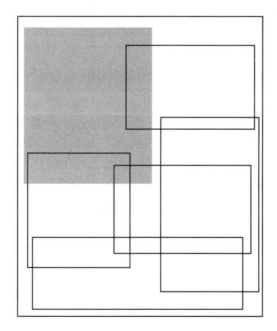

Fig. A.7. The Knowledge Hologram: A multifaceted image containing an unknown part.

holistic therapists are just as valuable to preventive medicine, helping patients avoid a relapse, whatever the syndrome may be. These two types of doctors must coexist, each looking to the other for whatever is missing in his or her method.

The body is a hologram. Four major functions, and only four, are found at the macro- and microscopic level. In terms of prevention, which is fundamental to any anti-aging program, or in terms of therapy, during and after a specific intervention, it is necessary to once again establish an optimal interaction among bodily functions.

> *"Logic leads to everything, as long as you can escape it."*
> ALPHONSE ALLAIS

GLOSSARY

aerobic: relating to or occurring in the presence of oxygen

alkaloid: chemical family of molecules, found in abundance in plants and responsible for some of their properties

anaerobic: relating to or occurring in the absence of oxygen

anti-aging: relating to a product or plan whose goal is to limit the damage related to the wearing down of cells, tissues, and organs associated with age

antigen: specific marker-protein of a virus, bacteria, or cell

apoptosis: programmed cell death

ATP: adenosine triphosphate, a molecule produced during the aerobic respiration cycle that is the energy source for all molecular and mineral movements at the cellular level

autoimmunity: inappropriate immune reaction in which an external antigen (bacteria, virus, food), after passing through the blood, generates an immune reaction against itself and against the cells from which it originated

base: substance capable of accepting or neutralizing hydrogen ions, which thereby raises a solution's pH; a purine or pyramidine group in a nucleotide or nucleic acid

benzopyrene: carcinogenic molecule generated by overcooking food

calcium EAP: chelated calcium-2-aminoethanolphosphate, also known as colamine phosphate, a cell membrane sealant approved in Germany for the treatment of multiple sclerosis

cameline: plant from the cruciferous family with a lipid extract containing high levels (30 percent) of polyunsaturated omega-3 fatty acids

carcinogen: substance capable of inducing cancer over the long term

carcinogenesis: process by which a cancerous lesion is induced in tissues and/or organs

catabolism: destructive metabolism; the breakdown of complex molecules in living organisms to form simpler ones, together with the release of energy

catabolized: transformed by the catabolic degradation process

central nervous system: designates the brain in its entirety and the spinal cord, in relation to the peripheral nervous system and the nerves

chelation: operation that consists of attaching to, and trapping, a chemical body (heavy metals) in order to eliminate it

cis: isomeric fatty acid shape in which double bonds form an angle; this is the active, fluid, biologically available, and easy-to-assimilate form of a fatty acid

clogging: process of gradual buildup of inert, nonassimilative molecules or incompletely broken down waste within the cell

CNRS: National Center for Scientific Research (France)

collagenases: enzymes that break the chemical bonds between the molecules of collagen, the main protein of connective tissue, which, when overstimulated, can cause fibrosis, the formation of excess fibrous connective tissue

combustion: biochemical operation that results in the destruction of a molecule by way of an oxidative process

cyclophosphamide: anti-cancer chemotherapy molecule that acts directly upon the DNA

cytokines: signaling proteins such as interferon and interleukins

cytoplasm: area of the cell between the nucleus and the cell membrane

destabilization: phenomenon that occurs when the DNA molecule is attacked, which results in the partial opening of the double chain of nucleotides in several places

DHA: decosahexanoic acid, a long-chain fatty acid found in abundance in fish oil

DHEA: a hormone produced by the adrenal gland and by the nervous system cells in our brain; it is a good marker of biological age

differentiation: process of cell specialization, beginning with a stem cell precursor

DNA: deoxyribonucleic acid, the long molecule found in the nucleus of the cell or the mitochondrion that is the seat of biological memory

dolomite: sea sediment, rich in calcium, magnesium, and several trace elements, most often in organic form

dopamine: neurotransmitter produced primarily in the brain, whose depletion in certain areas of the brain leads to Parkinson's disease

dry residue: the mineral content in water, measured after evaporation at a temperature of 180°C (356°F)

ectoderm: first layer of embryonic stem cells, which will produce, subsequent to embryonic development, all the central and peripheral nervous system cells

EDTA: ethylene diamine tetracetate, a synthetic amino acid chelating agent used to help remove primarily lead and cadmium from the body (but it is not a good chelator of mercury), best administered by injection, with very limited value as an oral agent

electrolyte: charged chemical body; positive/negative electric charge carrier

ELF: extremely low frequency; used in reference to electromagnetic waves

EM: electromagnetic

emunctory: organ (kidney, liver) or tissue (intestinal mucous membrane) whose function is to eliminate bodily waste

endoderm: second layer of stem cells produced by the ectoderm; it creates all of the mucous membranes throughout the body as well as the exocrine glands (such as the pancreas) and endocrine glands (such as the thyroid and thymus)

endoplasmic reticulum: flattened network of cytoplasmic cavities, surrounded by a membrane and protein synthesis areas that functions especially in the transport of materials within the cell and that is studded with ribosomes in some places

energy: motor behind all biochemical and biophysical bodily operations, in the form of electricity, magnetism, heat, or molecular chemical bonds, such as adenosine triphosphate

enzyme: protein necessary to complete biochemical reactions within a cell

EPA: ecosapentanoic acid, a long-chain polyunsaturated fatty acid of the omega-3 family found in fish

epithelium: mucous membrane cell line marking the border between two areas; able to secrete mucous (intestinal epithelium) and hormones (thyroid epithelium)

ferritin: protein carrying an iron atom and released en masse when a tissue is destroyed

free radicals: unstable chemical radicals created in mitochondrial aerobic respiration and normally neutralized by enzymes like SOD and GP

gamete: male or female germinal cell, that is, sperm or ovum

gene: particular segment of a DNA molecule, responsible for specific functions in the cell (such as the production of an enzyme, pigment, and so on)

germinal: holds within it the seed for future development; germinal cells are cells stemming from the ovum and sperm

gliadin: protein family found in grains of wheat and many other cereals, the quantity and diversity of which has increased sevenfold between 1920 and 2000, which may be the reason for several digestive intolerances among today's consumers

glutathione: tripeptide molecule (consisting of the three amino acids: cysteine, glutamate, and glycine) that is the major intracellular antioxidant; it also functions as a heavy metal chelator and detoxifier

glycation: protein, sugar, and oxygen interaction; source of AGE (advanced glycated end) products, serious factors in the aging of all tissues

Golgi body: group of flattened membrane disks found in the cellular cytoplasm and derived from the endoplasmic reticulum that digest and excrete numerous metabolites

hippocampus: area of the brain essential to learning and memory; an area of cerebral stem cell creation

histone: protein support, serving as a matrix to the DNA molecule

hologram: three-dimensional image reproduced from a pattern of interference produced by a split beam of coherent light, in which each component reflects the whole (see also appendix, "Holograms and Holography")

IGF1: insulin growth factor 1, a growth factor produced by the liver that is the principal marker for human growth hormone (HGH) activity

immunoglobulin: proteins of high molecular weight present in the serum and cells of the immune system that function as antibodies; they are classified in several categories: A, E, G, and M immunoglobulins (designated IgA, IgE, IgG, and IgM)

insulin: anabolizing hormone, produced by small beta-cell cellular islands in the pancreas

intolerance: inability of the body's enzymes to fully break down food or a molecule; the products of this incomplete breakdown most often produce inflammation, particularly intestinal inflammation

intoxification: impregnation of a tissue or an entire body by toxins, stemming from either a bacteria or disrupted tissue metabolism

in vitro: activity begun or created in the laboratory, in a test tube or Petri dish

in vivo: activity begun or created in a living body: vegetal, animal, or human

ion: negatively (anion) or positively (cation) charged atom

Krebs cycle: cycle of optimal oxygen usage in the cell involving the burning or oxidation of glucose to form energy-rich ATP molecules; named for the first person to describe it

lectin: food-based protein able to connect to intestinal (or other tissue) mucous membrane cell receptors, which can lead to inflammation or strong bodily agglutination

lymphoid: cell or tissue derived from connective tissue and in charge of immune function

lysosome: vesicle (derived from the endoplasmic reticulum) present in the cellular cytoplasm that is able to absorb foreign bodies (such as molecules, bacteria, viruses, and so on) and to digest them using enzymes

mesenchyme: tissue line derived from embryonic mesoderm; source of connective tissue that ensures the interweaving of all tissues and organs

mesoderm: third embryonic layer in order of appearance, which develops around the spinal cord and specifically forms the connective tissue, the blood, the vessels, the bones, and the muscles

methylation: biochemical attachment of a methyl radical ($-CH_3$) to another molecule in order to neutralize a poison (hepatic detoxification) or form another molecule for many possible functions, such as making a specific neurotransmitter or hormone

mitochondrion: organelle present within the cytoplasm that is the site of aerobic respiration, during which a glucose molecule is broken down by oxygen into water and adenosine triphosphate (ATP)

multipotent: in reference to a stem cell, able to transform into various cell types and thus to ensure over time very different functions

mutagenesis: appearance of a mutation in DNA characterized by a change in one or more of the bases (purine or pyrimidine) that make up the DNA

nitrous oxide: very well-known tissue transmitter produced by the body from an amino acid, arginine, whose properties include the regulation of vascular and smooth muscle tonicity and an anti-inflammatory action

nucleotide: basic unit in the DNA or RNA chain consisting of a specific sugar, a base (purine or pyramidine), and a phosphate (such as adenosine triphosphate)

nutritherapy: short- and long-term therapeutic strategy that aims to progressively reestablish normal bodily functioning through food selection on the one hand and micronutrient supplements (vitamins, minerals, trace elements, amino acids, and so on) on the other

Oncotest: test developed by Mirko Beljanski that measures the growth of carcinogenic DNA; used to determine if a substance is carcinogenic or has anti-cancer properties

organelle: a class of small organs or structures present in the cytoplasm of every cell (such as mitochondria, endoplasmic reticulum, and lysosomes)

parenchymas: the functional parts of the organs

peptide: short polymers of linked amino acids

peroxidation: formation of peroxides from a molecule (protein, fatty acid, sugar) via the attachment of an oxygen atom to an unstable double biochemical bond

peroxisome: organelle present in the cellular cytoplasm that encloses specific enzymes, bringing about molecular oxidation but also the neutralization of peroxidized derivatives (H_2O_2)

Petri dish: plastic dish containing a nutritive medium; used in laboratories for cell or microorganism cultures

pH: the logarithm of the concentration of hydrogen ions (H+) in a solution; value calibrated on a scale of 0 to 14, acids having a pH below 7 and bases having a pH above 7; ideal blood pH is 7.2

phospholipid: lipid (fatty substance) bound to phosphorus

plasticity: a tissue or cell's capacity to change shape

polarized: said of a cellular membrane that has different interior and exterior charges (because of an excessive external charge, which causes the difference in potential between the inside and outside)

polyamines: polypeptides, or protein remnants with more than one amino group, created during the breakdown of large proteins by various enzymes; useful in small numbers for stimulating the multiplication and maturation of normal tissues; harmful in large quantities, paralyzing cellular immunity and favoring cancerous growth

polymers: large molecules composed of repeating structural units, such as DNA and proteins

prebiotics: soluble fibers that are the preferential nutrients among probiotic bacteria, like bifidum

primer RNA: RNA molecule segment able to initiate cell division by attaching to a DNA

prion: abnormal protein that is able to replicate itself in large quantities in the cell until it pervades it and causes its death by asphyxiation; the prion acts like an infectious element and is transmitted from one host to another, and quite often even between two different species of hosts

probiotics: several types of bacteria that reside in the colon and are beneficial to the host (such as acidophilus); so-called friendly bacteria

provirus: virus without its protein envelope, which is written into cellular DNA in order to force it to produce copies of the original virus

qi gong: literally means "energy work," a practice composed of small gestures and various breathing techniques, with the goal of improving energy flow in the body, thereby improving health

receptor: DNA or membrane site, most often dealing with a protein able to connect to a specific hormone or a transmitter in order to activate an internal chain of reactions

reduction: addition of electrons (the smallest negatively charged particles) to a substance, atom, or molecule, an operation essential to all molecular and cell (re)construction

ribonuclease: enzyme that catalyzes the breakdown of RNA; capable of selecting an RNA at specific sites, enabling the cell to use RNA primers for new multiplications; in the case of cancer, this process must immediately be halted

ribosome: basic organelle in protein synthesis; rich in tRNA (transfer RNA), organized in a regrouped continuum, and attached to the external membrane of the granulous reticulum; able to read messenger RNA from the nucleus for protein transcription

RNA: ribonucleic acid, produced by the DNA in the nucleus (*nuclear RNA* or *n*RNA), in the cytoplasm (ribosomal RNA), and in the form of *messenger* (*m*RNA) and *transfer* (*t*RNA) RNA; also capable of influencing DNA duplication (primer RNA)

RNA fragment: partial section of an RNA, capable of action as important as priming bone marrow stem cell division

saturated: fatty acid molecule that does not have a double bond

serotonin: transmitter produced by the brain and in the intestine by the amino acid tryptophan

somatotropin: growth hormone (GH) produced by the anterior pituitary gland; responsible for growth in childhood, and in adults is involved in maintaining tonicity and body mass; it is indirectly involved in activation of other hormones, like insulin

stem cell: cellular originator of a tissue line, such as bone marrow stem cells that create blood cells; in an embryo only a few days old, the cells making up the three fundamental layers are called embryonic stem cells because they are totipotent

sterolic: said of a molecular nucleus whose structure is identical to those in the sterolic family

supplementation: additional micronutrients or hormones used to supplement a diet deemed deficient, or in the case of hormonal levels requiring a correction

synapse: junction between two neurons; when one neuron secretes a neurotransmitter, it crosses the synapse, attaches to a receptor on the adjoining neuron, and promotes an electrical discharge or nerve impulse down the second neuron

tai chi chuan: Chinese martial art expressed through slow movements and breathing techniques, allowing for optimal energy flow in the body

teralene: toxic molecule resulting from cooking; particularly common in everyday cooking fat

totipotent: in reference to a stem cell, able to transform into all cell types found in the body and thus to ensure all functions over time

trans: rigid fatty acid isomer that no longer has the fluidity or assimilability of the *cis* form; found in large amounts when unsaturated fatty acids are hydrogenated; trans fats are harmful to the body

transmitter: action molecule of a tissue, whose attachment to a receptor leads to a physiological action (for example, a neurotransmitter like noradrenaline, or a hormone like thyroxin)

tubule: long proteins that ensure the weaving of the cellular cytoplasm

unsaturated: said of a double or triple biochemical bond capable of attaching to one or several hydrogen atoms

Wi-Fi: wireless Internet connection that uses a network of electromagnetic waves, relayed by transmitting and receiving antennas

NOTES

INTRODUCTION: FROM DNA
TO OPTIMAL FUNCTIONING

1. "Prévenir les mécanismes du vieillissement," *Nutranews* (July/August 2001): 1–10.
2. For an extended explanation of a hologram, please refer to the appendix.
3. C. G. Nordau and Monique Beljanski, *A Pioneer in Biomedicine* (New York: EVI Liberty Corp., 2001).
4. Mirko and Monique Beljanski, *La santé confisquée,* 4th edition (Paris: Editiones Guy Trédaniel, 2003).
5. A. Berkaloff et al., *Biologie et physiologie cellulaires,* vols. 1–4 (Paris: Hermann, 1977).
6. Ibid.
7. www.ornl.gov/sci/techresources/Human_Genome/project/info.shtml#draft
8. Hervé Janecek, "Médecine traditionnelle chinoise et hologrammes: Un nouveau modèle de physiologie," lecture given at AFA Nantes conference in 1997 and AMAC Clermont-Ferrand in September 2004.
9. Ibid.
10. Ibid.
11. Ibid.

CHAPTER 1. EXTERNAL PROTECTION, ASSIMILATION, AND ELIMINATION

1. BioSante Pharmaceutical, *Recueil des conférences 2003* (Monpellier, France: Edition Adevi, 2003).

2. Jean-Philippe Moulinoux and Véronique Quemener, *Les polyamines,* Collection Médecine-Sciences (Paris: Flammarion, 1991).

3. Jean Seignalet, *L'alimentation ou la troisième médecine,* 5th edition (Paris: François Xavier de Guibert, 2004).

4. Peter D'Adamo, *Eat Right for Your Type,* New York: Putnam, 1996.

5. "Pour chasser la fatigue et retrouver toute votre énergie," *Nutranews* (October 2003): 2–7.

6. Institut Européen de Diététique et Micronutrition (IEDM), *La Micronutrition du cerveau seminar,* 2004.

7. Jean Seignalet, *L'alimentation ou la troisiéme médecine,* 5th edition (Paris: François Xavier de Guibert, 2004).

8. A very light mineral content is one with a dry residue of less than 100 mg/liter.

9. Robert Masson, *Diététique de l'expérience* (Paris: Guy Trédaniel, 2003).

10. Institut Européen de Diététique et Micronutrition (IEDM) newsletter no. 2 (2002/2003): 8, 19.

CHAPTER 2. INTERNAL STRUCTURE AND DEFENSE

1. "Heal Thyself: Patients' Bone Marrow Cells Restore Failing Hearts," American Heart Association Scientific sessions 2003 report (November 10, 2003). "Growth Factor Grows Stem Cells That Help Heal Hearts," American Heart Association Scientific sessions 2003 report (November 11, 2003). Both articles appeared in *Stem Cell Research News* 5, no. 22 (November 21, 2003): 1–3.

2. C. G. Nordau and Monique Beljanski, *A Pioneer in Biomedicine* (New York: EVI Liberty Corp., 2001).

3. Monique Beljanski, *Mirko Beljanski: Chronique d'une "fatwa" scientifique,* ed. Guy Trédaniel (Paris: Broché, 2003).

4. C. G. Nordau and Monique Beljanski, *A Pioneer in Biomedicine* (New York: EVI Liberty Corp., 2001).

5. Ibid.

6. A. Goyenvalle, A. Vulin, F. Fougerousse, F. Leturcq, J. C. Kaplan, L. Garcia, and O. Danos, "Rescue of Dystrophic Muscle through U7 snRNA-mediated Exon Skipping," *Science Express* (November 4, 2004), *Science* 306, no. 5702 (December 3, 2004): 1796–99, cited by J. Y. Nau, "Un espoir pour les myopathes," *Le Monde* (November 6, 2004).

7. "Heal Thyself: Patients' Bone Marrow Cells Restore Failing Hearts," American Heart Association Scientific sessions 2003 report (November 10, 2003). "Growth Factor Grows Stem Cells That Help Heal Hearts," American Heart Association Scientific sessions 2003 report (November 11, 2003). Both articles appeared in *Stem Cell Research News* 5, no. 22 (November 21, 2003): 1–3.

8. RNA fragments and other Beljanski products, as well as a list of medical professionals familiar with the Beljanski approach, can be obtained from Natural Source International, Ltd., 150 East 55th Street, 2nd Floor, New York, NY 10022 USA. Toll-free: (888) 308-7066; phone: (212) 308-7066; fax: (212) 593-3925. E-mail: info@natural-source.com; website: www.natural-source.com.

9. The identities of the individuals cited in the case studies have been changed to protect their medical records.

CHAPTER 3. ENERGY PRODUCTION AND DISTRIBUTION

1. A. Berkaloff et al., *Biologie et physiologie cellulaires,* vols. 1–4 (Paris: Hermann, 1977).

2. EA Pharma, Oligothérapie division, "Le stress oxydatif: Son implication en pathologie," Medical information letter from Laboratoires des Granions (2002).

3. "Acétyl-L-carnitine et acide alpha-lipoïque," *Nutranews* (September 2002): 1–6.

4. Thierry Schmitz, "La méthylation," *Pratiques de santé*, no. 3 (January 2004).

5. Bernard Friguet, "Stress oxydatif, protéines et vieillissement," *La Journée de la longévité* (June 21, 2003).

6. C. G. Nordau and Monique Beljanski, *A Pioneer in Biomedicine* (New York: EVI Liberty Corp., 2001).

7. Ibid.

8. Monique Beljanski, personal communication, December 18, 2003.

CHAPTER 4. COORDINATION AND MEMORY

1. Fred Gage, "Le cerveau en réparation," *Pour la Science,* no. 317 (March 2004): 77–81.

2. A. Berkaloff et al., *Biologie et physiologie cellulaires,* vols. 1–4 (Paris: Hermann, 1977).

3. David Servan-Schreiber, *Guérir, le stress, l'anxiété, la depression sans medicament ni psychanalyse* (Paris: Robert Laffont, 2003).

4. Bernard Friguet, "Stress oxydatif, protéines et vieillissement," *La Journée de la longévité* (June 21, 2003).

5. Françoise Clavel-Chapelon et al., "Breast Cancer Risk in Relation to Different Types of Hormone Replacement Therapy in the E3N-EPIC Cohort," *International Journal of Cancer* 114, no. 3 (April 10, 2005): 448–54.

6. "La débat sur la DHEA: Une revue critique des données expérimentales et cliniques," *Nutranews* (June 2004): 18–23.

7. Bruno Lacroix, "Favoriser sa production d'hormone de croissance," *Nutranews* (October 2002): 1–6.

8. E. von Zoch, *Thymus, Zentrale der Immunität,* 2nd edition (Heidelberg, Germany: Karl F. Haug Verlag, 1987).

9. "Entretien avec le Pr Vincent Castronovo," *Nutranews* (March 2003): 6–8.

CHAPTER 5. HEALING
DESTABILIZED DNA

1. Monique Beljanski, personal communication, December 18, 2003.

2. Françoise Clavel-Chapelon et al., "Breast Cancer Risk in Relation to Different Types of Hormone Replacement Therapy in the E3N-EPIC Cohort," *International Journal of Cancer* 114, no. 3 (April 10, 2005): 448–54.

3. C. G. Nordau and Monique Beljanski, *A Pioneer in Biomedicine* (New York: EVI Liberty Corp., 2001).

4. Jean Seignalet, *L'alimentation ou la troisième médecine,* 5th edition (Paris: François Xavier de Guibert, 2004).

APPENDIX: HOLOGRAPHY AND
HOLOGRAMS

1. K. H. Pribram, *Languages of the Brain* (Englewood Cliffs, N.J.: Prentice-Hall, 1971).

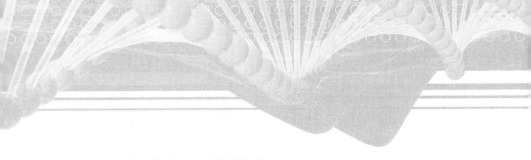

BIBLIOGRAPHY

REFERENCE WEBSITES TO SUPPLEMENT READING

www.beljanski.com

French and English website dedicated to Mirko Beljanski's work and its applications in biology and medicine.

www.canhelp.com

Website of CanHelp, a lifesaving alternative and complementary cancer treatment organization located in Livingston, N.J., that has been helping people with cancer since 1993 by tailoring information and resources to each patient's individual needs.

www.csif-cem.org

French website dedicated to the subject of extremely low-frequency (ELF) pollution.

www.genomics.energy.gov

Website that details the findings of the Human Genome Project, the international effort undertaken by the U.S. Department of Energy, to identify the 20,000 to 25,000 human genes and make them accessible for further biological study.

www.schachtercenter.com

Website of the Schachter Center for Complementary Medicine in Suffern, New York, a holistic health care institution providing alternative treatments for cancer and other illnesses.

www.sciencemag.org

Website for *Science* magazine.

www.stemcellresearchnews.com

Website that summarizes news regarding current stem cell research.

www.worldwildlife.org

Informational website for the World Wildlife Fund; contains many articles on environmental pollution and contamination.

BIBLIOGRAPHIC REFERENCES
(IN ENGLISH, FRENCH, AND GERMAN)

"Acétyl-L-carnitine et acide alpha-lipoïque." *Nutranews* (September 2002): 1–6.

"L'acide R lipoïque." *Nutranews* (December 2002): 12–14.

"Approche naturelle du TDAH Trouble de déficience de l'attention/hyperactivité par Bruno Lacroix." *Nutranews* (February 2004).

Beljanski, Mirko. "Radioprotection of Irradiated Mice—Mechanisms and Synergistic Action of WR-2721 and RLB." *Deutsche Zeitschrift für Onkologie* 23, no. 6 (1991): 155–59.

Beljanski, Mirko, and Monique Beljanski. *La santé confisquée.* 4th edition. Edited by Guy Trédaniel. Paris: Broché, 2003.

Beljanski, Mirko, Monique Beljanski, Christian Marcowith, and Hervé Janecek. *Cancer: L'approche Beljanski.* New York: EVI Liberty Corp., 2007.

Beljanski, Mirko, et al. "RNA Fragments (RLB) and Tolerance of Cytostatic Treatments in Hematology." *Deutsche Zeitschrift für Onkologie* 23, no. 2 (1991): 33–35.

Beljanski, Monique. "Lettre ouverte à la presse." CIRIS: Beljanski Foundation (August 2002). Published on www.beljanski.com.

———. *Mirko Beljanski: Chronique d'une "fatwa" scientifique.* Edited by Guy Trédaniel. Paris: Broché, 2003.

Berkaloff, A., et al. *Biologie et physiologie cellulaires.* Vols. 1–4. Paris: Hermann, 1977.

BioSante Pharmaceutical. *Recueil des conférences 2003.* Monpellier, France: Edition Adevi, 2003.

Borek, Carmia. "In the News: Fish and N-3 Fatty Acids Reduce Risk of Alzheimer's Disease." *Life Extension Magazine* (November 2003).

Cenacchi, T., et al. "Cognitive Decline in the Elderly: A Double Blind, Placebo-Controlled Multicenter Study on Efficacy of Phosphatidylserine Administration." *Aging* 5, no. 2 (1993): 123–33.

Chambon, Philippe, and Marie Beuzard. "Cancer les vraies raisons d'une épidémie." *Science et Vie* (June 2004): 46–69.

Chervet, Sophie. *Enquête sur un survivant illegal: L'affaire Gérard Weidlich.* Edited by Guy Trédaniel. Paris: Broché, 2002.

Clavel-Chapelon, Françoise, et al. "Breast Cancer Risk in Relation to Different Types of Hormone Replacement Therapy in the E 3N-EPIC Cohort." *International Journal of Cancer* 114, no. 3 (2003): 448–54.

"Combattre la dépression par des suppléments nutritionnels naturels." *Nutranews* (October 2004): 12–18.

D'Adamo, Peter. *4 groupes sanguins, 4 modes de vie.* Canada: Michel Lafon, 1999.

———. *Eat Right for Your Type.* New York: Putnam, 1996.

"La débat sur la DHEA: Une revue critique des données expérimentales et cliniques." *Nutranews* (June 2004): 18–23.

EA Pharma, Oligothérapie division. "Le stress oxydatif: Son implication en pathologie." Medical information letter from Laboratoires des Granions (2002).

"Entretien avec le Dr. Corinne Skorupka." *Nutranews* (July 2004): 2–7.

"Entretien avec le Pr Vincent Castronovo." *Nutranews* (March 2003): 6–8.

Ferreira, Fernanda M., et al. "Diabetes Induces Metabolic Adaptations in Rat Liver Mitochondria: Role of Coenzyme Q and Cardiolipin Contents." *Molecular Basis of Diseases* 1639, no. 2 (2003): 113–20.

Friguet, Bernard. "Stress oxydatif, protéines et vieillissement." *La Journée de la longévité* (June 21, 2003).

Gage, Fred. "Le cerveau en reparation." *Pour la Science,* no. 317 (March 2004): 77–81.

Gindin, J., et al. *The Effect of Plant Phosphatidylsérine on Age-Associated Memory Impairment and Mood in the Functioning Elderly.* Kaplan Hospital Rehovot, Israel: Geriatric Institute for Education and Research, 1995.

Goyenvalle, A., A. Vulin, F. Fougerousse, F. Leturcq, J. C. Kaplan, L. Garcia, and O. Danos. "Rescue of Dystrophic Muscle through U7 snRNA-mediated Exon Skipping." *Science Express* (November 4, 2004), *Science* 306, no. 5702 (December 3, 2004): 1796–99, cited by J. Y. Nau, "Un espoir pour les myopathes," *Le Monde* (November 6, 2004).

"Growth Factor Grows Stem Cells That Help Heal Hearts." American Heart Association Scientific sessions 2003 report (November 11, 2003). In *Stem Cell Research News* 5, no. 22 (November 21, 2003).

"Heal Thyself: Patients' Bone Marrow Cells Restore Failing Hearts." American Heart Association Scientific sessions 2003 report (November 10, 2003). In *Stem Cell Research News* 5, no. 22 (November 21, 2003).

Institut Européen de Diététique et Micronutrition (IEDM). La Micronutrition du cerveau seminar, 2004.

Institut Européen de Diététique et Micronutrition (IEDM) newsletter no. 2 (2002/2003): 8, 19.

Jacobs, Howard T., et al. "Premature Ageing in Mice Expressing Defective Mitochondrial DNA Polymerase." *Nature,* no. 429 (2004): 417–23.

Janecek, Hervé. "Médecine traditionnelle chinoise et hologrammes: Un nouveau modèle de physiologie." Lecture given at AFA Nantes conference in 1997 and AMAC Clermont-Ferrand in September 2004.

Lacroix, Bruno. "Favoriser sa propre hormone de croissance." *Nutranews* (October 2002): 1–6.

Lance, Pierre. *Savants maudits, chercheurs exclus.* Paris: Guy Trédaniel, 2003.

Lee, John R. *What Your Doctor May Not Tell You About Menopause: The Breakthrough Book on Natural Progesterone.* New York: Warner Books, 1996.

Lefeuvre, Jean-Claude. "La qualité de l'eau distribuée en France analyse critique." Presentation for the World Wildlife Fund (May 17, 2000).

Masson, Robert. *Diététique de l'expérience.* Paris: Guy Trédaniel, 2003.

Masson, Robert. *Super régénération par les aliments miracles.* Paris: Albin Michel, 1987.

Moulinoux, Jean-Philippe, and Véronique Quemener, eds. *Les poly-amines.* Collection Médecine Sciences. Paris: Flammarion, 1991.

Nicholson, Garth L. "Lipid Replacement as an Adjunct to Therapy for

Chronic Fatigue, Anti-Aging and Restoration of Mitochondrial Function." *Journal of the American Nutraceutical Association* 6, no. 3 (2003): 22–28.

Nordau, C. G., and Monique Beljanski. *Beljanski: A Pioneer in Biomedicine: Concepts, Theories, and Applications.* New York: EVI Liberty Corp., 2001.

"Numéro hors série le corps humain et son histoire." *Science et Vie* (March 2004).

Petitjean, Gérard. "Quand la chimie nous rend malade." *Le nouvel Observateur* 2082 (2004).

PiLeJe, Laboratoire de fondateur de Micronutrition "Les intolérances aux aliments et aux souches de la flore intestinale." *La Gazette* 1 (2003).

"Pour chasser la fatigue et retrouver toute votre énergie." *Nutranews* (October 2003): 2–7.

"Prévenir les mécanismes du vieillissement." *Nutranews* (July/August 2001): 1–10.

Pribram, Karl H. *Languages of the Brain.* Englewood Cliffs, N.J.: Prentice-Hall, 1971.

Quinton, René. *L'eau de mer, milieu organique.* Paris: Encre, 1995.

Rombi, Max. *Acides gras oméga 3 et anti-oxydants: De la fluidité des membranes cellulaires à la thérapeutique de l'avenir.* France: Romart, 1995.

Rueff, Dominique. *La bible des vitamines et des suppléments nutritionnels.* Paris: Albin Michel, 2004.

Schmitz, Thierry. "La méthylation." *Pratiques de santé,* no. 3 (January 2004).

Seignalet, Jean. *L'alimentation, ou la troisième médecine.* 5th edition. Paris: François Xavier de Guibert, 2004.

Servan-Schreiber, David. *Guérir, le stress, l'anxiété, la depression sans medicament ni psychanalyse.* Paris: Robert Laffont, 2003.

Souccar, Thierry, and Jean-Marie Curtay. *Le programme de longue vie.* Paris: Seuil, 1999.

Souccar, Thierry, and Isabelle Robard. *Santé, mensonges, et propagande.* Paris: Seuil, 2004.

Souetre, E., et al. "5-Methoxypsoralen as a Specific Stimulating Agent of Melatonin Secretion in Humans." *Journal of Clinical Endocrinology & Metabolism* 71 (1990): 670–74.

South, James. "Aging and Immunity." *International Antiaging Systems.* Available online at www.antiaging-systems.com/extract/entropy.htm, accessed September 12, 2008.

"Le traitement naturel de la depression." *Nutranews* (November 2001): 1–5.

Ward, Dean. "Le rôle des métaux lourds dans les maladies et le vieillissement." *Nutranews* (July 2003): 2–4.

Weil, Jean-Claude, and Miroslav Radman. "How Good Is Your Genome?" *The Royal Society* (October 2003).

West, Michael D. "Back to Immortality: The Opportunities and Challenges of Therapeutic Cloning." *Life Extension* (November 2003): 63–70.

WWF Detox Campaign. *Chemical Check Up: An Analysis of Chemicals in the Blood of Members of the European Parliament.* World Wildlife Fund report, April 2004.

Zoch, E. von. *Thymus, Zentrale der Immunität.* 2nd edition. Heidelberg: Karl F. Haug Verlag, 1987.

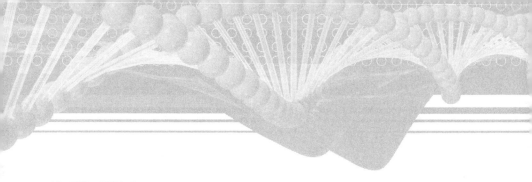

INDEX

Page numbers in *italics* refer to figures and charts.

ABOUT THE AUTHORS

DR. HERVÉ JANECEK is a clinician and biologist who specializes in nutrition, organotherapy, phytotherapy, and traditional Chinese medicine. Since 1990, he has presented his work in conferences all over the world. His topics have included therapeutic strategies applied to degenerative disorders and preventive medicine.

MONIQUE BELJANSKI studied biology and bacteriology before undertaking research in the field of molecular biology with her husband, the late Mirko Beljanski. This research continued for more than 20 years at the Pasteur Institute. She worked for 10 years at the Faculty of Pharmacology in France and is retired from the National Center of Scientific Research in France. She is currently the president of the Beljanski Foundation (www.beljanski.com).

BOOKS OF RELATED INTEREST

Decoding the Human Body-Field
The New Science of Information as Medicine
by Peter H. Fraser and Harry Massey with Joan Parisi Wilcox

Biogenealogy: Decoding the Psychic Roots of Illness
Freedom from the Ancestral Origins of Disease
by Patrick Obissier

The Biogenealogy Sourcebook
Healing the Body by Resolving Traumas of the Past
by Christian Flèche

Radical Medicine
Cutting-Edge Natural Therapies for a Toxic Age
by Louisa L. Williams, D.C., N.D.

Vibrational Medicine
The #1 Handbook of Subtle-Energy Therapies
by Richard Gerber, M.D.

Awakening the Energy Body
From Shamanism to Bioenergetics
by Kenneth Smith

Profound Healing
The Power of Acceptance on the Path to Wellness
by Cheryl Canfield

Alchemical Healing
A Guide to Spiritual, Physical, and Transformational Medicine
by Nicki Scully

INNER TRADITIONS • BEAR & COMPANY
P.O. Box 388
Rochester, VT 05767
1-800-246-8648
www.InnerTraditions.com

Or contact your local bookseller